Aids to Undergraduate Surgery

For Tracy and Victoria

For Churchill Livingstone:
Commissioning Editor: Laurence Hunter
Project Editor: Dilys Jones
Copy Editor: Teresa Brady
Production Controller: Debra Barrie
Sales Promotion Executive: Douglas McNaughton

Aids to Undergraduate Surgery

Peter M. Mowschenson

MRCP FRCS FACS

Clinical Assistant Professor, Harvard Medical School;
Surgeon, Beth Israel Hospital, Boston, Massachusetts, USA

FOURTH EDITION

CHURCHILL LIVINGSTONE
EDINBURGH LONDON MADRID MELBOURNE NEW YORK AND TOKYO 1994

CHURCHILL LIVINGSTONE
Medical Division of Longman Group Limited

Distributed in the United States of America by
Churchill Livingstone Inc., 650 Avenue of the
Americas, New York, N.Y. 10011, and by
associated companies, branches and
representatives throughout the world.

First edition 1978
Second edition 1983
Third edition 1989
Fourth edition 1994
  Reprinted 1995

ISBN 0-443-04966-1

British Library Cataloguing in Publication Data
A catalogue record for this book is available from
the British Library.

Library of Congress Cataloging in Publication Data

Mowschenson, Peter M.
  Aids to undergraduate surgery/Peter M.
Mowschenson. — 4th ed.
    p.   cm.
  Includes index.
  ISBN 0-443-04966-1
  1. Surgery—Outlines, syllabi, etc. I. Title.
  [DNLM: 1. Surgery—outlines. WO 18 M963a
1994]
RD37.3.M68 1994
617—dc20
DNLM/DLC
for Library of Congress   93-34955
                                               CIP

Produced by Longman Singapore Publishers Pte Ltd
Printed in Singapore

The
publisher's
policy is to use
**paper manufactured
from sustainable forests**

Contents

Contents

Preface

This fourth edition of *Aids to Undergraduate Surgery* continues the tradition of attempting to summarize the more important aspects of general surgery for the student. The book is aimed towards the best students by including topics and details an average undergraduate student might not be expected to know. Hopefully less informed students will be prompted to read further about subjects they find unfamiliar and the best students will find this book an educational aid.

Boston 1994   P.M.M.

1. Fluids and electrolytes

ANATOMY OF BODY WATER

70 kg man (ml)	Space	% of body weight
3 500	Plasma	5
10 500	Interstitial fluid	15
28 000	Intracellular fluid	40
42 000	Total body fluid	60 males
		50 females

APPROXIMATE VOLUME AND ELECTROLYTE CONTENT OF GASTROINTESTINAL FLUIDS

	Vol (ml)	Na	K	Cl	HCO₃ (mmol/l)
Gastric	1500–2000	60	10	120	0–25
Pancreatic	500–1000	140	5	75	80
Bile	300–1000	148	5	100	35
Small bowel	1000–3000	110	5	100	30
Diarrhoea	500–17 000	120	25	90	45

SODIUM

Predominant extracellular cation. Normal dietary intake 50–90 mmol/day. With normal renal function, urine sodium loss can be reduced to <1 mmol/day in face of salt restriction (aldosterone effect).

Hyponatraemia

Causes
1. Water overload
   a. Most commonly excess i.v. fluid administration
   b. Inappropriate ADH release

  (i) Head injury
  (ii) Morphine
  (iii) Barbiturates
  (iv) Carcinoma, e.g. lung
2. Addison's disease – chronic adrenal insufficiency

Complications
1. Convulsions
2. Stupor
3. Irrationality
4. Coma

Treatment
1. Water restriction
2. Severe cases may require partial correction with 3% saline infusion, especially in cases of coma
3. Steroids for Addison's disease

Hypernatraemia

Causes
1. Water deprivation
2. Loss of water in excess of electrolytes

Complications
1. Delirium
2. Hyperthermia
3. Renal failure

Treatment
Rehydration

POTASSIUM

Predominant intracellular cation. Normal dietary intake 50–100 mmol/day. Urine excretion a function of distal tubular exchange involving Na^+ and H^+. Daily replacement approx. 80 mmol

Hyperkalaemia

Causes
1. Renal failure
2. Trauma
3. Acidosis

Complications
1. Heart block
2. Diastolic arrest: more likely if $K^+ > 7$ mmol. (ECG changes: shortened QT interval, P waves peaked)

Treatment
1. Immediate: 80 mmol Na lactate/bicarbonate
2. 100 ml 50% dextrose with 10 units insulin i.v.
3. Cation exchange resin
4. Dialysis

Hypokalaemia  $\downarrow K^+$

Causes
1. Excess renal losses
   (i) Diuretics
   (ii) Hyperaldosteronism
   (iii) Cushing's disease
   (iv) Compensation for alkalosis (acid loss) induced by excess vomiting
2. Gastrointestinal losses

   (i) Diarrhoea
   (ii) Fistulae
   (iii) Vomiting (see above)

Complications
1. Muscle weakness and lethargy
2. Ileus
3. Cardiac arrhythmias. (ECG changes: S–T segment depression and T wave flattening)
4. Digitalis sensitivity

Treatment
1. Prevent: adequate daily replacement
2. Oral or intravenous replacement. Intravenous infusion of solutions containing more than 30 mmol/l can cause severe discomfort and subsequent phlebitis unless given via central line

CALCIUM

Mostly stored in bone. Dietary intake of 1–3 g daily. Urine excretion of approx. 300 mg/day, remainder in faeces

Hypocalcaemia

Causes
1. Following surgery for hyperparathyroidism or bilateral thyroid operations

2. Acute pancreatitis
3. Hypoparathyroidism
4. Malabsorption syndromes
5. Pancreatic and small bowel fistulae
6. Massive soft tissue infections
7. Severe magnesium depletion

Complications
1. Numbness and tingling: perioral, fingers and toes
2. Hyperreflexia. Positive Chvostek's sign
3. Abdominal and muscle cramps
4. Increased Q–T interval on ECG
5. Tetany. Hyperventilation is the most common cause of tetany, and is due to a decreased ionized calcium and not to a decrease in total serum calcium
6. Convulsions

Treatment
1. 10 ml of 10% calcium gluconate i.v. as a bolus, and repeat as necessary.
2. Rebreathing expired air for hyperventilation cases

Hypercalcaemia
See hyperparathyroidism

MAGNESIUM

50% is stored in bone. Diet contains about 240 mg/day. Mostly excreted in the stool, some in urine. Serum level is not a true reflection of body magnesium

Hypomagnesaemia

Causes
1. Starvation
2. Malabsorption
3. Protracted gastrointestinal fluid loss
4. Pancreatitis
5. Conn's syndrome (hyperaldosteronism)
6. Chronic alcoholism
7. Burns
8. Prolonged i.v. infusion without magnesium supplements

Complications
Same as hypocalcaemia

Treatment
Give 1.2 g MgSO$_4$ (equivalent to 240 mg Mg) i.v./day to patients liable to become deficient

Hypermagnesaemia

Causes
1. Chronic renal failure
2. Excess antacid therapy with Mg salts in patients with renal failure

Complications
ECG changes of hyperkalaemia

Treatment
Correct acidosis and volume depletion

WATER BALANCE

Intake
1. Normal adult oral intake: 2000–2500 ml
2. Water of metabolism: 200 ml

Output

1. Sensible
    (i) Urine   800–1000 ml
    (ii) Stool   200 ml
    (iii) Sweat   0–4000 ml/day depending on temperature elevation
    (iv) Drains, e.g. nasogastric tube

2. Insensible
    (i) Lungs
    (ii) Skin   12 ml/kg/24 hours

Third space loss
Translocation of extracellular fluid into peritoneum, bowel, tissues, etc. following trauma, e.g. surgery, sepsis, inflammation. Fluid remains extracellular, but is 'lost', since it does not participate in normal exchange with other fluid compartments. This fluid is recaptured as the patient recovers. The diuresis which results is referred to as 'mobilization of the third space'

Replacement of fluid and electrolytes
1. Review the prior 24 hours input and output record

2. Note patient's weight. (Patients normally lose ¼–½ lb/day on i.v. fluids)
3. Replace:
   (i) Measured losses
      Gastrointestinal losses with normal saline. See table, p. 1
      Urine output with 5% dextrose. Normal output is about 1000 ml/day. If patient is mobilizing third space this will increase urine output. However only a normal urine volume of 1000 ml should be replaced or a vicious cycle will be set up
   (ii) Insensible losses
      12 ml/kg/24 h with 5% dextrose
      Add extra for fever
   (iii) Predict third space losses. Depends on type of surgery, and disease. Normally cease 24–36 h after surgery, but may begin later if complications set in
   (iv) Potassium: give 60 mmol/day basic requirement. Add 30–40 mmol/l to normal saline being given to replace gastro-intestinal losses (e.g. nasogastric tube)

The careful measurement and recording of intake, output, and daily weight will be the best guide to fluid replacement.
Haematocrit and electrolyte measurements are indicated in patients having rapid fluid shifts. Once the patient is stable they are required much less frequently

PARENTERAL FEEDING

The vast majority of patients undergoing surgery have adequate energy reserves, and can withstand the catabolic period of surgery without intravenous feeding and its attendant complications

Relative indications
1. Patients with severe malnutrition requiring major surgery, e.g. long-standing oesophageal stricture with profound weight loss
2. Patients with postoperative complications leading to delayed return of oral feeding, e.g. prolonged partial small bowel obstruction, enteric fistulae
3. Patients with prolonged sepsis and renal failure who are severely catabolic and require surgery
4. Patients with short bowel syndrome following extensive resection, e.g. Crohn's disease

Complications
1. During insertion of the central line
   Pneumothorax
   Haemothorax
   Cardiac tamponade
   Stroke

Thoracic duct injury
Air embolism
2. Sepsis (bacterial/fungal). Patients on combined steroid and antibiotic therapy at greatest risk
   a. line
   b. solution
3. Hyperosmolar states
4. Hypo-/hypernatraemia
5. Calcium/magnesium disorders
6. Fatty acid deficiency − linoleic acid
7. Hyperammonaemia
8. Reactive hypoglycaemia
9. Acidosis
10. Zinc deficiency − acrodermatitis, hair loss
11. Copper deficiency − leukopaenia, lymphocytosis
12. Chromium deficiency − diabetes, polyneuropathy

ACID–BASE ABNORMALITIES

1. Respiratory acidosis − resulting from hypoventilation
   (i) Acute
      a. Narcotics
      b. Head injury
   (ii) Chronic
      Chronic obstructive airway disease
2. Respiratory alkalosis − resulting from hyperventilation
   (i) Anxiety/pain
   (ii) Mechanical ventilation
3. Metabolic acidosis
   (i) Widened anion gap acidosis
      a. Shock with anaerobic metabolism
      b. Excess aspirin ingestion
   (ii) Normal gap acidosis
      a. Diarrhoea
      b. Pancreatic fistula
4. Metabolic alkalosis
   (i) Excess loss of acids
      Vomiting
   (ii) Gain in bicarbonate
      a. Diuretics
      b. Antacids

2. Shock

DEFINITION OF SHOCK

Shock is defined as a severe physiological abnormality associated with diminished tissue perfusion

TYPES

Hypovolaemic shock

Physiology
  1. Diminished intravascular volume and venous return
  2. Fall in cardiac output and blood pressure
  3. Increased peripheral vascular resistance (alpha receptor)
      (i) Splanchnic
      (ii) Renal
      (iii) Pulmonary
      (iv) Skin

Causes
  1. Internal/external bleeding
  2. Other fluid losss

Septic shock

Physiology
  1. Toxin release – most commonly Gm negative organisms
  2. Cardiac output is elevated
  3. Peripheral vascular resistance is low
  4. Oxygen extraction is reduced

Causes
  1. Urinary tract
      (i) Pyelonephritis
      (ii) Catheterization
      (iii) Instrumentation

2. Pneumonia
3. Wound infections
4. Abscesses, e.g. pancreatic, subphrenic
5. Central lines

Cardiogenic shock

Physiology
1. Heart failure
2. High filling pressures
3. Low cardiac output
4. Elevated peripheral vascular resistance aggravates problem by increasing afterload

Causes
1. Postmyocardial infraction
2. Following open heart surgery

Irreversible shock
(i) Persistent loss of fluid from vascular compartment
(ii) Red and white cells aggregate in stagnant capillaries forming microthrombi
(iii) Disseminated intravascular coagulation (DIC) is initiated

CELL METABOLISM

1. Lactic acid accumulation – anaerobic metabolism
2. Decrease in ATP production – anaerobic metabolism
3. Membrane function
   (i) Sodium leaks into cells; potassium leaks out of cells
   (ii) Lysosomes fragment – autodigestion
4. Fatty acid mobilization
   (i) Ketonaemia
   (ii) Fat emboli to lung

ORGAN FAILURE

1. Kidneys – acute tubular necrosis
2. Lungs – adult respiratory distress syndrome
3. Gut – ischaemia due to low flow state, e.g. gastric stress ulceration

TREATMENT

1. Prevent – identify high risk patients early
2. Diagnosis of underlying cause

3. Correction of hypovolaemia. May require placement of central monitoring catheter (e.g. Swan–Ganz catheter)
4. Correction of acid–base/electrolyte abnormalities
5. Antibiotics
6. Pressors. Depending on the clinical situation and measurements obtained from central monitoring devices, haemodynamic situation can be improved by judicious choice of pressor agents. Depending on the pressor and dose used, the effect can be to increase or decrease regional blood flow
7. Neutralize gastric pH. It has been shown that antacids/histamine receptor antagonists can reduce the incidence of bleeding from gastric erosions
8. Surgery
   (i) Stop bleeding
   (ii) Drain pus
   (iii) Remove dead bowel
   (iv) Intra-aortic balloon pump for cardiogenic shock
9. Appropriate ventilator support
10. Dialysis for renal failure
11. Treatment of DIC

3. Burns

DEPTH OF BURN

1. Partial thickness – heal within 3 weeks with good epithelial coverage
   (i) 1° burn – erythema
   (ii) Superficial 2° burn
2. Deep 2° burns – heal with unsatisfactory skin coverage; require the same treatment as full thickness burns
3. Full thickness – total destruction of all epithelial remnants

CLINICAL DIFFERENTIATION OF BURN DEPTH

Burn biopsy, vital dyes, thermography, etc. have all been used to increase clinical accuracy of differentiating burn depth, but are unreliable

1. Superficial 2° burn
   (i) Painful and sensitive to pin prick
   (ii) Surface is moist and hyperaemic
   (iii) Blanches on pressure
2. Deep 2° burns and full thickness injury
   (i) Insensitive to pin prick
   (ii) Surface is dry and white
   (iii) No blanching on pressure

LOCAL EFFECTS OF BURN

1. Pain, swelling, loss of function
2. Loss of fluid electrolyte, protein
3. Infection: may convert partial thickness burns to full thickness. Gram positive organisms, e.g. staph/strep colonize wounds early. Gram negative organisms, e.g. *Pseudomonas* lead to invasive wound sepsis mostly after 5 days
4. Thrombosis, esp. thermal and electrical burns

SYSTEMIC EFFECTS

1. Cardiovascular effects

   (i) Generalized increase in capillary permeability with loss of intravascular volume: 50% of plasma volume can be lost within 3 hours of a 40% burn

   (ii) Haemolysis. Rate proportional to amount of 3° burn

2. Respiratory failure
   (i) Upper airway obstruction secondary to inhalation injury or facial trauma
   (ii) Lower airway obstruction or parenchymal lung damage secondary to:
      a. Inhalation of toxic combustion products
      b. Fluid overload during resuscitation
      c. Sepsis

3. Catabolism is increased by:
   (i) Resetting of the hypothalamic regulatory mechanism and increased catecholamines leading to increased BMR
   (ii) Heat loss — if environment is cool
   (iii) Sepsis
   (iv) Complications, e.g. renal/respiratory failure

4. Gastrointestinal changes
   (i) Ileus — may be a manifestation of unrecognized sepsis
   (ii) Haemorrhage. 80% of patients with 40% burns have gastric erosions predominantly involving the fundus in first 3 days following a burn. Minority of these patients proceed during the ensuing days to develop major gastric/duodenal ulcer (Curling's) which may bleed or perforate. Stomach is more common site but 15% have both
   (iii) Focal ischaemic intestinal necrosis
   (iv) Colonic pseudo obstruction
   (v) Acute acalculous cholecystitis
   (vi) Duodenal obstruction in patients who have much weight loss secondary to compression of duodenum by superior mesenteric artery

5. Immunosuppression. Extent depens on burn size. Particularly marked in patients with >50% burns

ESTIMATION OF BURN SURFACE AREA

Rule of nines
(Unreliable in children because limbs are relatively smaller)

Head and neck	9%
Each arm	9%
Each leg	9 × 2%
Front of trunk	9 × 2%
Back of trunk	9 × 2%
Perineum	1%

GENERAL MANAGEMENT

1. Ensure adequate airway; Tracheostomy best avoided to reduce risk of infection. May require bronchoscopy to assess degree of airway injury
2. Fluid resuscitation. Different formulae are all designed to maintain organ perfusion with least possible infused volume; and are only a guide to management. Infusion is modified according to:
   (i) Hourly urine output − > 0.5 ml/kg/hour
   (ii) Haematocrit
   (iii) Acid−base status, electrolytes
   (iv) Central venous monitoring − all lines carry a risk of introducing infection.
   Patients must be treated individually. Peripheral lines must be changed frequently to avoid phlebitis
3. Sedation and pain control.
4. Tetanus prophylaxis
5. Antibiotics used if infection sets in
6. Antacid therapy to reduce incidence of gastric erosions
7. Nutrition: give orally whenever possible. Intravenous feeding with high protein solutions has been shown to be of benefit in major burns
8. Psychological support. Extremely important
9. Rehabilitation: early mobilization of extremities

LOCAL MANAGEMENT OF BURNS

Much depends on site and extent of the burn, individual patient, personal preference, and policy of different burn units. Open methods tend to be used on large areas which are difficult to dress; closed methods for small burns and burns of the extremities

1. Escharotomy
   (i) Circumferential burns may impede the circulation
   (ii) Doppler may be used to detect a distal pulse
   (iii) Chest wall movements may also be restricted by eschar
2. Debridement
   Wet to dry dressings till eschar has been removed, and underlying granulation tissue is suitable to receive a graft
3. Excision of burn
   Major advantage of excision is to reduce recovery time
   (i) Risks
       a. Blood loss
       b. Converting 2° areas to full thickness
       c. Risk of introducing infection
       d. Hazards of anaesthesia
   (ii) Indications
       a. Small full thickness burns
       b. Removal of persistent eschar

      c. Treatment of focal areas of infection
      d. Debridement of high voltage electrical injuries
      e. Deep 2° burns on dorsum of hand
      f. Staged excision of extensive burns in young patients
4. Prevention of infection
  (i) Topical agents
      a. Sulfamylon cream (mafenide acetate):
         (i) Very effective against *Pseudomonas* and Gram negative organisms
        (ii) Carbonic anhydrase inhibitor – leads to metabolic acidosis
      b. Silvadene cream (silver sulphadiazine):
         (i) Causes less pain on application
        (ii) Less effective against *Pseudomonas* and other Gram negative organisms
  (ii) Isolation beds, sterile technique
 (iii) Effective debridement
 (iv) Frequent i.v. site changes
  (v) Biological dressings
      a. Viable cutaneous allografts
         (i) Prevent wound desiccation
        (ii) Promote formation of granulation tissue
       (iii) Limit bacterial proliferation
       (iv) Decrease protein and red cell loss
        (v) Decrease pain
       (vi) Protect exposed tendons, nerves, and vessels
      b. Cutaneous xenografts – less successful
      c. Bilaminate membrane with collagen-based dermal analogue and tissue culture-derived epithelial cells is a new develoment which will become increasingly important
5. Autografts
  (i) Sheet grafts with careful attention to expressing subgraft fluid collections
  (ii) Mesh grafts
      a. Used if shortage of donor sites
      b. Minimize subgraft collections
      c. Closed dressings can be used, which can reduce need for external fixation devices
6. Maintenance of function
  (i) Eyes – protect cornea
  (ii) Limbs – joint motion
 (iii) Ears – pressure necrosis of cartilage

FEATURES OF ELECTRICAL BURNS

1. Tissue is damaged as a result of conversion of electric to thermal energy
2. Damage occurs along the route taken between entry and exit sites

3. Misleadingly small cutaneous burns may overlie larger area of damaged muscle and deep tissues. Fluid resuscitation has to be carefully considered in view of this
4. Early decompression of muscle compartments may be required
5. A variety of neurological changes can be seen affecting the central and peripheral nervous system
6. Gastrointestinal injury is unusual, but liver necrosis, pancreatitis, intestinal perforation, etc. have all been reported

4. Malignant disease in general

MORTALITY FROM CANCER

In decreasing frequency

Men	Women
Lung	Breast
Colon/Rectum	Colon/Rectum
Prostate	Uterus
Pancreas	Lung
Stomach	Ovary

AETIOLOGY OF MALIGNANT DISEASE

1. Chemical, e.g.
   (i) Smoking – lung cancer
   (ii) Asbestos – mesothelioma
2. Physical
   (i) X-rays – leukaemia
   (ii) Ultraviolet light – skin cancer
3. Viral
   EB virus – Burkitt's lymphoma
4. Genetic, e.g.
   Familial polyposis coli
5. Miscellaneous
   Geographical, diet

SPREAD OF MALIGNANT DISEASE

1. Direct extension, e.g. longitudinal growth of oesophageal cancer
2. Lymphatic, e.g. especially carcinomas
3. Vascular, e.g. especially sarcomas and carcinomas
4. transcoelomic, e.g. stomach

CLINICAL MANIFESTATIONS

Effect of primary tumour
1. Expansive growth, e.g. obstruction, lump
2. Infiltrative growth, e.g. pain from nerve involvement, fixation of tumours
3. Necrosis – bleeding/infection

Effect of metastases
1. Lymphadenopathy (compression of adjacent structures)
2. Lung (dyspnoea)
3. Liver (jaundice)
4. Brain (epilepsy)
5. Skin (nodules)
6. Bone (fractures)

Systemic manifestations
1. Cachexia, weight loss, anaemia, fever
2. Cutaneous, e.g. acanthosis nigricans (lung, stomach), dermatomyositis
3. Haematological, e.g. polycythaemia (kidney, cerebellum)
4. Vascular, e.g. thrombophlebitis (lung, pancreas)
5. Hormonal and metabolic, e.g.
   (i) Cushing's – lung
   (ii) ADH secretion – lung
   (iii) Hypercalcaemia – lung, breast, myeloma
   (iv) Hypoglycaemia – liver
6. Gout – lymphomas
7. Neuromuscular, e.g.
   (i) Cerebellar degeneration – lung
   (ii) Myasthenia gravis – thymus

DANGER SIGNALS OF CANCER

1. Change in bowel or bladder habit
2. Non-healing sore
3. Unusual bleeding or discharge
4. Breast lump or other growing lump
5. Dysphagia
6. Obvious change in wart or mole
7. Persistent cough or hoarseness
8. Loss of weight or appetite
9. Bleeding or discharge from any body orifice or from nipple

PRINCIPLES OF MANAGEMENT

Diagnosis
1. History, physical examination

2. Appropriate investigation
3. Biopsy and staging

General treatment options
1. No treatment, e.g. incurable elderly patient
2. Surgery alone, e.g. basal cell carcinoma
3. Surgery and radiation therapy, e.g. seminoma
4. Radiation alone, e.g., stage I/II Hodgkin's
5. Chemotherapy, e.g., stage IV Hodgkin's
6. Radiotherapy, chemotherapy and surgery – Wilm's tumour
7. Immunotherapy – experimental

Surgical procedures
1. Wide local excision, e.g. basal cell carcinoma
2. Radical local excision, e.g. malignant melanoma
3. Radical local excision with en bolc node dissection, e.g. radical mastectomy
4. Extensive procedures, e.g. pelvic exenteration for recurrent cervical cancer
5. Surgery for recurrent cancer, e.g. obstruction following bowel resection
6. Resection of metastases, e.g., liver, lung
7. Palliative surgery, e.g. colostomy, gastrojejunostomy

5. Radiation therapy

MECHANISM OF ACTION

Radiation causes ionization of water in cells. The hydroxy and peroxide radicals which form cause DNA and chromosome disruption. Neoplastic cells are more sensitive.
RAD is unit of measurement, and expresses amount absorbed.
4500–6000 rads is lethal dose for most tumours

COMPLICATIONS

General
1. Malaise, nausea, vomiting
2. Pancytopaenia
3. Increased incidence of malignancy, e.g. leukaemia
4. Skin ulceration

Specific systems
1. Cardiovascular – pericarditis
2. Respiratory – pneumonitis amd fibrosis
3. Alimentary – bowel stricture, ulceration, perforation, fistula
4. Genitourinary – nephritis, gonadal atrophy
5. Central nervous – cerebral oedema, myelitis conjunctivitis and cataracts
6. Musculoskeletal – bone necrosis

EXAMPLES OF INDICATIONS FOR PALLIATIVE RADIOTHERAPY

1. Lung cancer
   (i) Intractable cough
   (ii) Superior vena cava obstruction
   (iii) Pathological fractures
   (iv) Pain
   (v) Haemorrhage
   (vi) Brain metastases

2. Oesophageal cancer
   Dysphagia
3. Breast cancer
   a. Bone pain
   b. Local recurrence
   c. Brain metastases

POSSIBLE ADVANTAGES OF PREOPERATIVE RADIOTHERAPY

1. Can reduce the bulk of tumour
2. May reduce fixation to surrounding tissues and thereby increase resectability
3. May decrease local recurrence rate
4. May increase cure rate

RELATIVE INDICATIONS FOR POSTOPERATIVE RADIOTHERAPY

1. Inadequate tumour margin following resection
2. Seminoma (periaortic and iliac nodes)
3. Wilm's tumour   ~e protozotou~
4. Medulloblastoma
5. Some cases of ovarian bladder, and lung cancer
6. Rectum – May be given in conjunction with adjuvant chemotherapy (5-FU) to reduce local recurrence rate.

6. Postoperative complications

PREOPERATIVE MEASURES TO REDUCE COMPLICATIONS

1. Identify risk factors for bleeding disorders, e.g. aspirin intake, prior history of bleeding
2. Reduce weight and stop smoking
3. Note any allergies and current use of drugs
4. Ensure that patients with pulmonary problems are in the best possible condition
5. Treat heart failure
6. Ensure adequate bowel preparation for colon surgery
7. Identify pre-existing infections, e.g. urinary
8. Identify predisposing factors for postoperative urinary retention
9. Ensure adequate preoperative fluid resuscitation to avoid postoperative renal failure

GENERAL CAUSES OF POSTOPERATIVE FEVERS

1. Atelectasis – generally occurs within first 48 hours
   a. Predisposing factors
      (i) Obesity and smoking
      (ii) Wound pain
      (iii) Opiates and drowsiness
      (iv) Muscular weakness
      (v) Nasogastric tubes
      (vi) Abdominal distension
   b. Prevention
      (i) Stop smoking preoperatively
      (ii) Treat bronchitis preoperatively (bronchodilators, antibiotics)
      (iii) Deep breathing and coughing
      (iv) Incentive spirometry
      (v) Adequate analgesics, avoiding excess
      (vi) Treatment of established atelectasis may involve:
         a. Aggressive physiotherapy
         b. Nasotracheal suctioning
         c. Bronchoscopy to aspirate mucus

          d. Positive pressure ventilation
  2. Pneumonia
     a. May develop from atelectasis
     b. Aspiration. Supine posture, and absence of protective
        reflexes predispose to this. Special conditions also
        predispose:
        (i) Pregnancy
        (ii) Elderly
        (iii) Obese
        (iv) Bowel obstruction
        Measures to reduce aspiration include:
        (i) No oral intake for 6 hours prior to anaesthesia
        (ii) Preoperative gastric decompression for emergency cases
        (iii) Preoperative administration of antacids/H_2 blockers
        (iv) Cricoid pressure until intubation and cuff inflation is
             accomplished
  3. Wound infection. Streptococcal and clostridial wound infections
     may cause high fever and incisional pain within 24 hours of
     surgery. Most wound infections present later, e.g. 5 days
  4. i.v. phlebitis. Incidence can be lowered by changing sites every
     24–48 hours
  5. Urinary tract infections and prostatitis
  6. Deep venous thrombosis
  7. Central line sepsis
  8. Gout or pseudogout
  9. Parotitis
  10. Drug reaction
  11. Transfusion reactions
  12. Complications of specific operations, e.g. anastomotic leaks,
      subphrenic or pelvic abscess, mediastinitis, pericarditis

DEEP VENOUS THROMBOSIS

Predisposing causes
Virchow's triad:
  (i) Stasis
  (ii) Injury to vessel wall
  (iii) Hypercoagulable state

Incidence
Radioiodine-labelled fibrinogen scanning
  (i) 30% of patients have DVT following surgery
  (ii) 50% following hip fracture
  (iii) At least 50% many be clinically silent

Diagnosis
  1. Clinical – frequently inaccurate; 50% false – ve/ + ve rate

   (i) Calf vein thrombosis. May have minimal calf swelling.
      Homan's sign may be present
  (ii) Femoral vein thrombosis. Swelling is usually present in calf,
      along with tenderness in calf popliteal region, or adductor
      canal
 (iii) Iliofemoral thrombosis. Left leg more commonly involved:
      Pain, tenderness, and swelling usually seen. Can progress to
      phlegmasia cerulia dolens and gangrene
 (iv) Axillary vein thrombosis. Effort syndrome in muscular men.
      Swelling of the arm and tenderness over the vein.
2. Doppler
   (i) Good above level of mid-thigh – most effective at detecting
      major venous thrombosis
  (ii) Will not detect non-occlusive thrombus or occlusive
      thrombus if there are large collateral veins
3. Impedance plethysmography
   More reliable than Doppler method for femoropopliteal and calf
   vein thrombosis, but is best used to detect major venous
   thrombosis
4. Phlebography
   (i) Indicates extent and degree of fixity of thrombus
  (ii) Contraindicated in presence of peripheral vascular disease
 (iii) May be indicated in a patient with equivocal signs or
      symptoms, or with equivocal non-invasive studies

Prophylaxis
1. Early ambulation
2. Pneumatic boots
3. Subcutaneous heparin: 5000 units s.c. every 12 hours. It is
   important to give the first dose shortly before the operation
   The incidence of DVT is reduced to about 10%
4. Intravenous heparin or oral anticoagulants (warfarin) for patients:
   (i) With prosthetic valves
  (ii) Undergoing high risk operations, such as hip replacement
 (iii) With prior history of deep venous thrombosis
5. Intermittent dextran 70

PULMONARY EMBOLUS

Risk factors
1. Extensive trauma or surgery
2. Pregnancy
3. Elderly or obese patients
4. Splenectomy, hip or pelvic surgery
5. Malignant disease
6. Oestrogen therapy (birth control pills)

7. Previous deep venous thrombosis or pulmonary embolus
8. Myocardial infarction

Diagnosis
1. History
    (i) Pleuritic chest pain
    (ii) Haemoptysis
    (iii) Dyspnoea
    (iv) Syncope
2. Physical examination
    (i) Signs of DVT – the majority of pulmonary emboli occur without any signs of a DVT
    (ii) Pleural rub
3. Investigations
    (i) Arterial blood gas – 80% have lowered Pa,o_2
    (ii) Chest X-ray – may show wedge-shaped infarction, area of decreased vascularity, effusion
    (iii) Ventilation–perfusion lung scan
    (iv) Pulmonary arteriogram
    (v) ECG changes (S wave I; Q wave lead III; inverted T wave in lead III is classical)

Treatment
1. General, e.g. oxygen
2. Drugs
    (i) Intravenous heparin
    (ii) Oral anticoagulation
    (iii) Streptokinase
3. Mechanical
    (i) Various sorts of inferior caval devices which filter blood. These are indicated in patients who have a contraindication to anticoagulation, e.g. bleeding ulcer or who have ongoing pulmonary embolism despite full anticoagulation. Modern devices can be inserted percutaneously under X-ray guidance
    (ii) Operations to extract embolus are rarely performed

FAT EMBOLISM

Causes
1. Fractures, e.g. tibia, hip
2. Extensive trauma
3. Burns
4. Severe infection
5. Pancreatitis

Clinical features
1. Dyspnoea, hypoxaemia, cyanosis
2. Altered level of consciousness

3. Focal cerebral signs
4. Petechial haemorrhages – mainly in the upper part of the body – skin, fundi, mucosal surfaces
5. High fever

Diagnosis
1. Depends on a high degree of clinical suspicion since signs develop late
2. Earliest change is hypoxaemia
3. Chest X-ray shows scattered consolidation (snowstorm appearance)
4. Fat in:
   a. Sputum – unreliable
   b. Urine – in severe cases
   c. Blood – frozen section of whole blood for fat
5. Elevated lipase (exclude pancreatitis)

Treatment
1. Careful handling of fractures to prevent fat embolism
2. Oxygen
3. Ventilation with positive end expiratory pressure is most effective in severe cases
4. Use of steroids is controversial

TETANUS PROPHYLAXIS

General principles
1. Debride devitalized tissue
2. Remove foreign bodies
3. Do not close contaminated wounds
4. Antibiotics in select cases only, e.g. some rectal injuries or puncture wounds

Immunization

Clean wounds
1. Patients without prior immunization: 0.5 ml tetanus toxoid, followed by further doses at 6 and 12 weeks
2. Patients who have been previously immunized but have not received a booster within 5 years: 0.5 ml tet. tox.

Contaminated wounds
1. Patients without prior immunization or with no booster within 5 years: 250 units human immune globulin and 0.5 ml tet. tox. followed by the full course of immunization
2. Patients who have received a booster within 12 months require no further prophylaxis

INDICATIONS FOR PROPHYLACTIC ANTIBIOTICS

1. Patients at risk of subacute bacterial endocarditis, e.g. mitral valve disease, prosthetic valves
2. Patients undergoing prosthetic joint or vascular compontents.
3. Operations which involve contamination to some extent, e.g. colon or oesophageal resection

As a general rule prophylactic antibiotics should be given in the perioperative period and then dicontinued. Prolonged administration of antibiotics is accompanied by undesirable side-effects, e.g. the emergence of antibiotic-resistant organisms

CONDITIONS PREDISPOSING TO GAS GANGRENE

1. Extensive devitalization of muscle mass especially buttock, thigh, shoulder
2. Impaired arterial supply, e.g. arterial compression, injury
3. Contamination by soil or clothing
4. Criminal abortion
5. Puerperal infection
6. Diabetic foot
7. Gross contamination during bowel surgery

RISKS OF ANTIBIOTIC THERAPY

1. Allergic reaction. Can be lethal
2. Toxicity, e.g. ototoxicity with gentamicin
3. Development of resistant bacteria
4. Diarrhoea
5. Pseudomembranous colitis. Secondary to *Clostridium difficile* (treat with vancomycin or metronidazole)
6. Oral monilia

POSTOPERATIVE RENAL FAILURE

Oliguria/anuria in the postoperative period should be regarded as an emergency

Prerenal causes
Hypovolaemia is easily the most common cause
1. Haemorrhage
2. Uncorrected losses from vomiting, burns, peritonitis

Renal causes
1. Ususally follows uncorrected prerenal causes
2. May also be due to:
   (i) Incompatible blood transfusion
   (ii) Myoglobinuria in crush injuries

    (iii) Circulating nephrotoxins in sepsis
    (iv) Toxic drug levels, e.g. aminoglycosides

Postrenal causes
1. Catheter obstruction is the most common cause
2. Bladder injury or ureteric ligation may have to be considered as a cause depending on the type of surgery

7. Skin and subcutaneous tissues

SKIN LUMP

Examination
1. Position, shape, size, colour
2. Consistency, attachments, edge, surface
3. Tenderness, temperature
4. Pulsatility, bruit
5. Cough impulse
6. Transillumination
7. Regional lymph nodes

Sites for common skin problems
1. Sebaceous epidermoid cyst
   a. Scalp
   b. Ear lobule
   c. Back
   d. Scrotum
   e. Vulva
2. Ganglia
   a. Wrist
   b. Dorsum of foot
   c. Flexor aspect of fingers
   d. Peroneal tendons
3. Pilonidal sinus
   a. Vast majority occur posterior to the anus in the natal cleft
   b. Other sites include:
      (i) Axilla
      (ii) Umbilicus
      (iii) Amputation stump
      (iv) Between fingers
      (v) Genitalia

Nail bed lesion
Differential diagnosis:
1. Haematoma

2. Exostosis
3. Malignant melanoma
4. Glomus tumour

MALIGNANT LESIONS

Squamous cell carcinoma
1. Predisposing factors
   (i) Senile keratosis
   (ii) Bowen's disease
   (iii) Lupus vulgaris
   (iv) Ultraviolet and X-rays
   (v) Tar, soot, smoking
   (vi) Chronic ulceration, e.g. Marjolin's ulcer
   (vii) Immunosuppressive drugs
2. Sites: mostly in the head and neck region
3. Spread to lymph nodes

Basal cell carcinoma
1. 90% occur on the face especially around the nose, eyes, hairline
2. Typically have a rolled pearly edge with central ulceration
3. Sun exposure increases incidence
4. Treated by excision or superficial radiation
5. Rarely spread to lymph nodes

Marjolin's ulcer
1. Malignant change in an ulcer, scar, or sinus
2. Slow-growing
3. Painless
4. Slow lymphatic spread

PIGMENTED LESIONS

Indications for removal:
1. Any lesion undergoing change
2. Lesions in areas subject to trauma
3. Black moles greater than 0.5 cm in diameter especially on leg/back
4. Naevi on soles of feet, mucous membranes, genitalia
5. Moles in anxious patients with bad family history
6. Children with solitary growing mole
7. Moles causing cosmetic problems

MELANOMA

Classification
1. Intradermal melanoma or naevus – the common mole

2. Compound melanoma or naevus
3. Juvenile melanoma
4. Junctional melanoma
5. Malignant melanoma

Suspicious factors
1. Increase in size of lesion
2. Increase in pigment
3. Areas of depigmentation
4. Ulceration or bleeding
5. Irritation
6. Statellite lesions and spread of pigment from edge of lesion
7. Regional lymph node enlargement or distant metastases

Prognosis

1. Clark's classification

Level	Extension	% metastases	% 5-year survival
I	Epidermis only	0	100
II	Into papillary dermis	7	90
III	To papillary–reticular junction	42	88
IV	Into reticular dermis	53	60
V	Into subcutaneous fat	93	15

2. Breslow's classification

Level	Thickness (mm)	% metastases
I	< 0.76	0
II	0.76–1.50	25
III	> 1.50	60

3. Type of lesion
  (i) Superficial spreading melanoma – 70%
  (ii) Nodular melanoma – worse prognosis
  (iii) Lentigo maligna melanoma – most slow-growing

Treatment
1. Excision of primary melanoma
   (i) <0.76 mm   0.5 cm margin
   (ii) 0.76–1.5 mm   2 cm margin
   (iii) >1.5 mm   4 cm margin ± skin graft

2. Regional nodes
   a. Relative indications for elective regional lymph node dissection (removal of clinically uninvolved nodes draining the area of the primary). Evidence that elective regional lymph node excision benefits the patient is weak
      (i) If the primary is in the immediate vicinity of the nodes
      (ii) With large, ulcerated, rapidly growing lesions
      (iii) If histology of the primary reveals deep dermal or lymphatic involvement
   b. Contraindications to elective regional node dissection:
      (i) Primary with unpredictable drainage, e.g. back
      (ii) Primary far removed from the draining area, e.g. lower leg
      (iii) Slow-growing, flat, non-ulcerated primary
      (iv) Microscopically superficial lesion, e.g., level 1, < 0.76 mm
      (v) Patient in poor general health
   c. Therapeutic regional lymph node excision is the removal of clinically involved nodes. This is generally recommended in the absence of further spread
3. Excision of solitary metastases can sometimes be helpful.
4. Regional chemotherapy with melphalan and hyperthermia (40°C) under investigation
5. Radiation therapy – can sometimes alleviate pain
6. Immunotherapy, e.g. interleukin – under investigation

8. Head and neck

EXAMINATION OF HEAD AND NECK

1. Skin – scalp, face, neck
2. Mouth (remove dentures, use tongue depressor, good lighting)
    (i) Entire buccal mucosa
    (ii) Openings of Stenson's and Wharton's ducts
    (iii) Tongue (all surfaces)
    (iv) Floor of mouth
    (v) Tonsils or tonsilar bed
    (vi) Soft palate
    (vii) Hard palate
3. Neck
    (i) Larynx (indirect/fibre-optic laryngoscopy)
    (ii) Trachea
    (iii) Sternocleidomastoid muscle
    (iv) Lymph node areas (anterior and posterior triangles)
    (v) Salivary glands
    (vi) Thyroid
4. Structures misdiagnosed as cervical lymph nodes
    (i) Carotid bulb
    (ii) Tip of hyoid bone
    (iii) Posterior belly of the omohyoid
    (iv) Transverse process C2
    (v) Cervical rib
5. Sites which metastasize to cervical lymph nodes
    (i) Below and behind the ear. Nasopharynx
    (ii) Angle of mandible
        a. Submaxillary area
        b. Floor of mouth
        c. Tonsils
    (iii) Submental region
        a. Tip of tongue
        b. Lower lip
        c. Gingivobuccal sulcus
    (iv) Middle third of the neck
        a. Oropharynx

  b. Larynx
  c. Thyroid
  (v) Supraclavicular area
  a. Lung
  b. Mediastinum
  c. Breast
  d. Infradiaphragmatic source may spread to the left side (Virchow's node), e.g. stomach

FEATURES OF OROPHARYNGEAL CARCINOMAS

1. Predisposing factors
  (i) Smoking
  (ii) Alcohol
  (iii) Sunlight
  (iv) Syphilis
  (v) Predisposing factors
  (vi) Men > 50 years
Multiple sites may be at simultaneous risk for development of malignancy

2. Lip
  (i) Lower lip – 93%
  (ii) Upper lip – 5%
  (iii) Angle of the mouth – 2% – worse prognosis

3. Tongue
  (i) Tip/free border most frequently involved
  (ii) Palpation often reveals ulcer is 'tip of an iceberg'
  (iii) Lymph nodes involved in 40%, especially posterior 1/3 lesions
  Submental nodes from tip of tongue
  Submandibular nodes – from sides of tongue
  (iv) Posterior 1/3 lesions may present with pain referred to the ear

4. Tonsil
  (i) Often causes persistent sore throat
  (ii) Squamous cell carcinoma – 85%
  (iii) Lymphosarcoma – 15%

5. Nasopharynx
Differential diagnosis:
  (i) Hypertrophied lymphatic tissue (adenoids), or lymphoma
  (ii) Juvenile angiofibroma
  (iii) Rathke's pouch cyst – craniopharyngioma
  (iv) Dermoids

(v) Mixed tumours
(vi) Carcinoma
Symptoms:
    (i) Nasal stuffiness
    (ii) Deafness (blocked eustachian tubes)
    (iii) Epistaxis (especially angiofibroma)
    (iv) Dysphagia
    (v) Facial pain
    (vi) Spread of malignant disease can cause III, IV, V, VI, cranial
        nerve palsies
    (vii) This is a difficult area to examine and patients present late

6. *Maxillary sinus:*
  Symptoms:
    (i) Nasal discharge (bloody/purulent)
    (ii) Epiphora
    (iii) Facial swelling
    (iv) Proptosis
    (v) Diplopia
    (vi) Palatal ulceration

7. *Larynx*
  Must be excluded in every case of persistent hoarseness
  Differential diagnosis
    (i) Polyp
    (ii) Nodule
    (iii) Retention cyst
    (iv) Leukoplakia
    (v) Papillomas
  Treatment of laryngeal carcinoma
    (i) Limited to true cord – radiation
    (ii) Extending beyond true cord or recurring following X-ray
        treatment:
    (i) Laryngectomy (partial/total) ± radiation therapy
    (ii) Neck dissection is performed if lymph nodes are involved

TREATMENT OF OROPHARYNGEAL CARCINOMA

Great majority are squamous cell carcinomas
  1. Primary lesion
    (i) Radiation therapy – external beam, interstitial or peroperative
    (ii) Resection
  2. Regional lymph nodes – radical neck dissection if nodes clinically
    involved and no evidence of further spread
  3. Chemotherapy with agents such as bleomycin and cisplatin
    (i) Advanced disease
    (ii) Increasing use preoperatively, and in conjunction with
        radiation therapy

PAROTID GLAND

Examination of the parotid gland
1. Palpation of the gland
2. Test VII nerve
3. Palpate the regional lymph nodes
4. Visualize and compress the duct orifice
5. Palpate fauces for deep lobe involvement

Differential diagnosis of 'parotid' swelling
1. Parotid lesion
2. Sebaceous cyst
3. Lipoma
4. Lymph node
5. Adamantinoma
6. Neuroma of VII nerve

Parotid lesions
1. Tumours
   a. Mixed tumours
      (i) 90% occur in the parotid, mostly in the superficial lobe
      (ii) Recur if enucleated
      (iii) Can undergo malignant change
      (iv) Occur mostly in patients <50 years
   b. Adenolymphoma (Warthin tumour)
      (i) Present after 50 years age usually
      (ii) 10% are bilateral
      (iii) May feel cystic
   c. Carcinoma
      (i) Pain
      (ii) Rapid growth
      (iii) Lymphadenopathy
      (iv) VII nerve palsy
2. Parotitis
   (i) Mumps
   (ii) Postoperative and debilitated patients
   (iii) Chronic recurrent
   (iv) Calculi
3. Mikulicz's syndrome
   (i) Sarcoid
   (ii) Reticulosis
   (iii) Sjögren's syndrome
   (iv) TB

9. Thyroid disorders

PHYSICAL EXAMINATION

1. General inspection.
   - (i) Does patient appear hyper/hypo/euthyroid? (tremor, lid lag, exophthalmos)
   - (ii) Note voice, skin, hoarseness, stridor
2. Palpation
   - (i) Pulse – tachycardia, atrial fibrillation, tachycardia during sleep
   - (ii) Tracheal deviation?
   - (iii) Goitre: smooth/nodular? Movement on swallowing
   - (iv) Cervical lymph node enlargement
3. Auscultation
   Bruit of Graves' disease
4. Indirect laryngoscopy
   Exclude recurrent laryngeal nerve palsy

In the elderly hypo- and hyperthyroidism may have atypical presentations. Therefore always consider the diagnosis

INVESTIGATION OF THYROID DISEASE

1. Ultrasound determines whether a mass is solid or cystic
2. Needle biopsy – fine needle aspirate/core needle aspirate
3. Tests of activity:
   - (i) $^{123}I/^{99m}Tc$ scans for functional status
   - (ii) Total T3, T4
   - (iii) TSH
4. Detection of circulating antibodies
   - (i) Hashimoto's
   - (ii) Graves' disease
   - (iii) Spontaneous hypothyroidism
5. Calcitonin. May be raised in cases of medullary thyroid carcinoma or in response to provocative testing with pentagastrin/calcium infusion test. May be used to detect early cases of MEA II syndrome
6. Chest X-ray or CT scan of the neck and upper chest may need to be done to evaluate the airway prior to resection of large goitres, and also to assess substernal goitres

HYPERTHYROIDISM

Causes of hyperthyroidism
1. Toxic diffuse goitre of Graves' disease
2. Toxic multinodular goitre
3. Toxic adenoma
4. Artefacta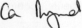

Eye signs of Graves' disease
1. Spasm of the upper lid
2. External ophthalmoplegia
3. Exophthalmos with proptosis
4. Supraorbital and infraorbital swelling
5. Congestion and oedema

Management of hyperthyroidism
1. Medical
    (i) Children and adolescents
    (ii) Pregnancy
    (iii) In preparation for surgery
2. Radioiodine (^{131}I)
    (i) Used for most patients except the above
    (ii) Patients who relapse following surgery
3. Surgery
    (i) Patients who have a strong aversion to radioiodine
    (ii) Patients who wish to have a rapid result, e.g. patients who want to become pregnant
    (iii) Patients with large glands/toxic adenomas
    (iv) Patients with marked eye symptoms – eye signs may be aggravated by radioiodine

Results
1. Medical
    (i) 30–50% success rate at 10 years – most patients require 2 years of treatment
    (ii) No means of predicting who will respond. Return of T3 suppressibility is a good index of inactivity
    (iii) Requires close co-operation of the patient
    (iv) Drugs can cause blood dyscrasias
2. Radioiodine
    60% incidence of hypothyroidism at 10 years and this continues to increase with time
3. Surgery (bilateral subtotal thyroidectomy)
    (i) Result is prompt
    (ii) Relapse rate of approx. 8%
    (iii) Hypothyroidism in approx. 8%
    (iv) Complications in experienced hands extremely low (<1%)

(v) Preparation for surgery:
   a. Correction of thyrotoxicosis, with antithyroid drugs followed by surgery, is most commonly used
   b. Beta blockers for 5–7 days alone is less common alternative
   c. Lugol's iodine 8–10 days preoperatively used to reduce vascularity of gland – benefit controversial

GOITRE

Control   *Cancer*
Compress   *Cosmetic*

Indications for surgery
1. Tracheal compression with respiratory problems
2. Dysphagia
3. Concern about the possibility of carcinoma
4. Retrosternal goitre especially if deviating the trachea
5. Prior history of irradiation to the head and neck (see below)

SOLITARY THYROID NODULE

Pathology
1. Approximately 10–20% of truly solitary thyroid nodules are malignant
2. 50% of patients with clinically solitary nodules are found to have multiple nodules by scan or at operation

Indicators of possible thyroid carcinoma
1. Family history of thyroid carcinoma
2. Histoy of prior low dosage radiation therapy to the head and neck for conditions such as acne, ringworm, thymic enlargement, tonsillitis. This was more commonly performed in the USA than in the UK. (Papillary thyroid carcinoma)
3. Solitary cold nodule – 10–20%
4. Accompanying laryngeal nerve palsy or Horner's syndrome
5. Regional lymphadenopathy
6. Positive/suspicious needle aspirate

THYROID CANCER

Prognosis
Prognosis better in patients <50 years, since well differentiated tumours with less malignant biological behaviour tend to be found

Types of thyroid carcinoma

Type	Incidence	Predominant age	Lymph	Bloodstream spread
Papillary	60–70%	Young <30	+ + +	+
Follicular	20%	Middle >30	+	+ +
Medullary	3–6%	Can be familial	+ +	+ +
Anaplastic	10–15%	Old	+ +	+ +

Treatment
1. Extent of operation depends on
   (i) Pathological type
   (ii) Distribution in gland
   (iii) Common surgical sense
   (iv) Personal prejudice. There is controversy regarding the need for total thyroidectomy. The disease tends to be indolent and well-designed long-term clinical trials are lacking
2. In summary:
   (i) Remove involved lobe and isthmus for unilateral low invasive disease, e.g. low grade follicular carcinoma
   (ii) Do total thyroidectomy for:
      a. Multicentric disease, e.g. papillary carcinoma or prior history of neck irradiation
      b. Familial cases of medullary thyroid carcinoma
      c. Operable anaplastic carcinoma
   (iii) Modified neck dissection if nodes are involved.
3. Postoperative radioiodine ^{131}I may be effective for some residual tumour, pulmonary or bone metastases
4. Lifetime replacement with thyroxine is essential following total thyroidectomy, and generally regarded as beneficial following less extensive operations, by suppressing TSH level which may stimulate tumour growth

THYROIDECTOMY

Complications
1. Recurrent laryngeal nerve palsy. Avoided by identification of the nerve and any extralaryngeal branches. Bilateral damage paralyses abductors of the vocal cords (posterior cricoarytenoids) causing airway obstruction. Unilateral damage causes a hoarse voice, but may become asymptomatic following compensation by the other cord
2. Superior laryngeal nerve palsy. Nerve supplies the cricothyroid muscle. Damage is much more common than recognized. Leads to inability to shout or reach high notes in singing

3. Pneumothorax. During resection of substernal goitres air may enter the mediastinum
4. Hypocalcaemia – secondary to parathyroid gland damage
5. Haemorrhage – presents with stridor and feeling of pressure. Requires immediate opening of incision and evacuation of haematoma
6. Thyroid storm – used to be quite common before patients were well prepared with antithyroid drugs, prior to surgery for Graves' disease
   (i) Hydrocortisone 100 mg i.v.
   (ii) Beta blockers
   (iii) Cooling blanket
   (iv) Large doses of Na or K iodide

NECK MASS

Differential diagnosis
1. Sebaceous cyst
2. Lipoma
3. Thyroid or parathyroid tumour
4. Cystic hygroma
5. Carotid artery aneurysm/carotid body tumour
6. Submandibular/parotid tumour
7. Pharyngeal pouch
8. Branchial cyst

[Handwritten annotations:]

Other – sebaceous cyst
lipoma
salivary gland
muscle tumour
neurofibroma
chemodectoma
laryngocoele
TB abscess

MID LINE
thyroglossal cyst
thyroid
dermoid cyst
submental LN.

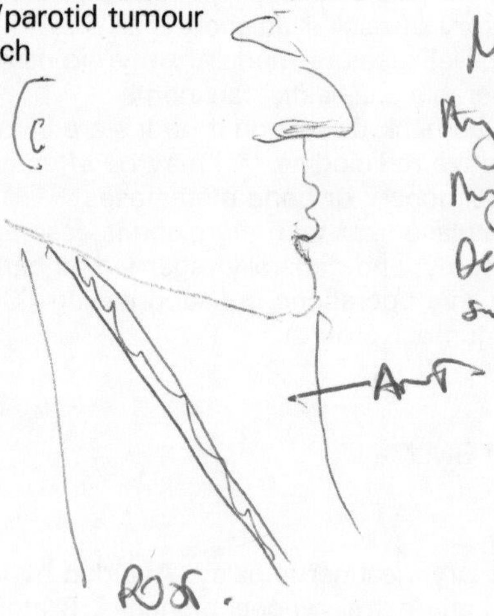

ANT

POST.

Ant. Δ – carotid aneurysm/body tumour
– branchial cyst
– sup./deep LN
– sternomastoid tumour
– submandibular gland tumour

Post Δ – pharyngeal pouch, subclavian aneurysm
cystic hygroma – cervical rib
– supraclavicular rib

10. Parathyroid

Ca   PO₄   Alk Ph

1°
2°   ↑(2)

HYPERCALCAEMIA

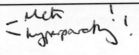

← Mets
← hyperparathy !

Differential diagnosis
1. Metastatic carcinoma to bone
2. Hyperparathyroidism
3. Multiple myeloma
4. Milk – alkali syndrome
5. Thiazide diuretics
6. Sarcoidosis
7. Vitamin D intoxication   *Vit D ↑*
8. Hyperthyroidism
9. Paget's disease
10. Familial hypocalcuric hypercalcaemia
11. Infantile hypercalcaemia

Treatment
1. Chronic – oral phosphate, low calcium diet
2. Acute
   (i) Rehydrate patient
   (ii) Induce a diuresis with saline and frusemide
   (iii) Mithromycin/calcitonin
   (iv) Steroids especially for hypercalcaemia, secondary to bone metastases

EMBRYOLOGY AND ANATOMY
1. Inferior glands
   (i) Arise from 3rd branchial pouch along with thymus
   (ii) Most lie near lower thyroid pole but 20% lie on or within suprasternal portion of the thymus
   (iii) May lie anywhere from mandible to anterior mediastinum
2. Superior glands
   (i) Arise from 4th branchial pouch
   (ii) Most lie adjacent to the cricothyroid notch close to the recurrent nerve

41

(iii) When ectopic they may lie in posterior mediastinum
3. Supernumerary glands occur in approx. 5% population

HYPERPARATHYROIDISM 1°.

Pathology
1. Single gland enlargement   80%
2. Multiple gland enlargement   20%
   (i) With renal failure
   (ii) MEA syndrome
   (iii) Familial hyperparathyroidism
   (iv) Rarities – cysts, carcinomas

Clinical features
1. Most cases are asymptomatic, and detected as a result of routine screening
2. Renal: stones, infection, nephrocalcinosis, polyuria
3. Bones: pain, fractures, cysts on X-ray —decalcified→ osteitis fibrosa cystica
4. Gastrointestinal: constipation, peptic ulceration, pancreatitis, increased incidence of gallstones, heartburn
5. General: lassitude, mental changes (may be severe especially in the elderly)

Investigation   stones, bones, abdo groans.
1. Exclude other causes of hypercalcaemia
2. PTH levels (intact hormone best)↑
3. Small parts ultrasound examination of the neck
4. Thallium-technetium scan
5. CT scan especially for mediastinum
6. Selective venous catheterization and PTH assays
7. Selective arteriograms

Localization studies are only required in patients who have undergone prior exploration. With an experienced surgeon primary neck exploration is 95% successful

Surgery
1. Aim is to identify 4 glands
2. Frozen sections identify parathyroid tissue, but not pathology, i.e. adenoma vs hyperplasia
3. Single gland enlargement – remove enlarged gland
4. Multiple gland enlargement – 3½ glands are removed, or total parathyroidectomy with autotransplant to forearm depending on personal preference

Complications of parathyroidectomy
1. Failure to recognize or remove the pathology
2. Recurrent nerve damage
3. Symptomatic hypocalcaemia (identical symptoms may be due to hypomagnesaemia)
4. Haemorrhage
5. Pseudogout — _pyrophat_
6. Pancreatitis — rare and mechanism unknown
7. Psychosis

↑ Ca⁺ — renal problem

↓ RT —

↑ PTH — ↑ PO₄ excret.

suppersected decalcefied
& cyst format.

↑ Ca⁺ resorption in
bones

↑ Ca ↑ excreted in urine
↑ PO₄

↑ Alk phosphatase

↓ PTH ↓ Ca — tetany (4.1.5mmol)

Trousseau sign ⎱ ↓ Ca⁺
Chvostek sign ⎰

11. Breast

BREAST DISEASE

Clinical presentation
1. Lump. Differential diagnosis:
    (i) Dominant mass which is subsequently shown to be composed of tissue with fibrosis, microcysts, adenosis, atypia: 'fibrocystic changes'
    (ii) Solitary cyst
    (iii) Fibroadenoma
    (iv) Cancer
    (v) Fat necrosis
    (vi) Lipoma
2. Pain – usually cyclical and worse premenstrually
    (i) Idiopathic – not significant
    (ii) Fibrocystic breast tissue
    (iii) Less commonly
        a. Costochondritis
        b. Abscess
        c. Carcinoma
        d. Superficial thrombophlebitis – Mondor's disease
3. Nipple discharge
    (i) Spontaneous uniductal bloodstained discharge
        a. 20–30% have an associated underlying malignancy
        b. Intraduct papilloma/carcinoma
        c. Duct ectasia
        d. Fibroadenosis with cysts
    (ii) Serous, e.g. during pregnancy
    (iii) Brown green, e.g., fibroadenosis
    (iv) Milky, e.g. following lactation/galactocoele
    (v) Purulent
   Note: discharges provoked by pressure are not significant.
4. Mammographic abnormality.
    (i) Mass
    (ii) Microcalcifications
    (iii) Skin thickening

LYMPHATIC DRAINAGE OF THE BREAST

1. Laterally to the axillary lymph nodes.
   - (i) Level I   Lateral to the lateral border of pectoralis minor
   - (ii) Level II   Behind the pectoralis minor
   - (iii) Level III   Medial to the pectoralis minor
2. Medially to the internal mammary nodes

BREAST CANCER

Staging (TNM)

T_0 No evidence of primary tumour
T_{is} Carcinoma in situ, Paget's disease
T_1 Tumour 2 cm or less in greatest dimension
T_2 Tumour greater than 2 cm but not more than 5 cm
T_3 Tumour more than 5 cm in greatest diameter
T_4 Tumour of any size extending to chest wall or skin
N_0 No regional lymph node metastases
N_1 Metastases to moveable ipsilateral axillary lymph nodes
N_2 Ipsilateral axillary nodal metastases fixed to one another or to other structures
N_3 Metastases to ipsilateral internal mammary nodes
M_0 No distant metastases
M_1 Distant metastases

Mammography

1. Screening for signs of malignancy in patients >35 years
   Impalpable breast cancers detected by mammography <1 cm (minimal breast cancer) are accompanied by a 5-year disease-free rate of 93% or greater.
2. Follow up of contralateral breast following mastectomy or both breasts following primary radiation treatment of breast cancer
3. Needle localization of impalpable breast masses or microcalcifications for biopsy
4. Ultrasound is sometimes useful in association with mammography to distinguish between impalpable solid/cystic lesions and evaluation of breasts which are dense and therefore not suitable for mammography
5. Mammography may not reveal up to 10% of breast cancers – therefore physical examination and mammography are complementary

Needle aspiration

1. Provides a rapid and inexpensive way of deciding if a palpable breast mass is solid or cystic
2. Breast cyst
   - (i) Aspirate should be clear or greenish brown. If fluid tests

positive for blood – biopsy
  (ii) There should be no residual mass following aspiration.
       Otherwise biopsy is indicated
3. Cytology. Positive result avoids the need for a separate biopsy
   and enables full discussion of alternative therapy with patient
   before operation. Negative result is not so helpful, but may be
   reassuring under certain circumstances, if correlated with the
   clinical findings and mammography. Several studies now indicate
   that a negative result may in fact be about 90% accurate, but
   the dictum that *a dominant breast mass must be biopsied* still
   stands.

Risk factors
1. Previous breast cancer
2. Genetic factors
     (i) History of maternal breast cancer increases the risk 2–3
         times in a patient. Normal incidence is 1:12
    (ii) Cancer occurs at a younger age and is more frequently
         bilateral in patients with + ve FH
3. Sex and hormonal milieu
     (i) Breast carcinoma in males account for < 1% cases
    (ii) Age of first pregnancy
   (iii) Breast feeding
    (iv) Early menarche
     (v) Late menopause
4. Biopsy indicating
     (i) Highly atypical hyperplasia
    (ii) Lobular carcinoma in situ
5. Age
     (i) Incidence increases with age
    (ii) Women at 85 years have twice the incidence of women 65
         years
6. Multiple ill-understood factors including
     (i) Blood type O in younger patients, type A in older patients
    (ii) Miscellaneous, e.g wet cerumen, diet

Clinical features
1. 80% are scirrhous adenocarcinomas
2. 50% occur in the upper outer breast quadrant
3. Starting from a single cell it takes 30 doubling times for a
   tumour to reach 1 cm in size. Therefore it may take 5 years for
   a tumour to become clinically palpable!
4. The chance of distant metastases is greater with axillary nodal
   involvement, and the number of nodes
5. Most common metastatic sites are:
     (i) Lung   65%
    (ii) Liver   56%

  (iii) Bones   56%
  6. Physical examination
    (i) Skin dimpling
   (ii) Nipple retraction
  (iii) Satellite skin lesions
  (iv) Oedema of the breast – peau d'orange
   (v) Dominant mass – irregular firm mass fixed/mobile
  (vi) Axillary or supraclavicular node enlargement
 (vii) Hepatomegaly
(viii) Pleural effusion
  (ix) Bone tenderness

Histological classification
1. Paget's disease of nipple
    (i) Presents as a scaling unilateral nipple lesion
   (ii) Always due to a ductal carcinoma which has invaded the
        skin. In 30% cases this is intraductal, and in the remainder
        invasive ductal cancer
  (iii) Any eczematous nipple lesion which persists must be
        biopsied to exclude Paget's disease
  (iv) Carries a better prognosis than other forms
2. Ductal carcinoma
    (i) Intraductal
   (ii) Invasive ductal (papillary, comedo, scirrhous, medullary,
        colloid, tubular, inflammatory)
3. Lobular carcinoma
    (i) In situ – marker for breast cancer. It is a histological finding
        indicating a particular patient may well have multicentric,
        bilateral, disease propensity. If followed non-operatively, such
        patients have an approx. 1% per year chance of developing
        invasive carcinoma. Some patients decide to have bilateral
        mastectomies, others decide to be followed closely
   (ii) Invasive
4. Rare forms of carcinoma, e.g. sarcoma

Treatment

1. *Local control of disease*
  a. Modified radical mastectomy ± reconstruction
     (i) Large tumour in small breast
    (ii) Extensive intraductal component in primary tumour –
         increased chance of local recurrence following radiation
   (iii) For patients who wish to avoid radiation or for whom
         radiation is inconvenient or deemed unsafe
   (iv) For patients with more than one cancer in a breast
    (v) If resection of the tumour requires removal of the nipple and
        areola

   b. Lumpectomy and node dissection followed by radiation therapy
      (i) Seems to be as effective in local control and cure as
          mastectomy in properly selected patients
      (ii) Extent of node dissection varies from 10 node sampling to
           'complete' dissection depending on institution and surgeon
   c. Advanced breast cancer $>T_3$ and inflammatory carcinoma may
      require radiation $\pm$ chemotherapy instead of or prior to surgery
   d. Reconstruction – immediate/delayed
      (i) Implant
      (ii) Flap
          a. Latissimus dorsi
          b. Rectus abdominis

2. *Adjuvant therapy*
   a. Chemotherapy appears beneficial in premenopausal women
      (i) With positive nodes
      (ii) Poor prognostic histological features, e.g. lymphatic/vessel
           invasion, poorly differentiated tumour,
      and postmenopausal women ER and PR – ve with + ve nodes
   b. Tamoxifen beneficial in postmenopausal women with ER + ve
      tumours

3. *Palliation of advanced breast cancer*
   a. Surgical
      (i) Excision of local disease to prevent/treat ulceration
      (ii) Relief of complications, e.g. pathological fractures
   b. Radiation
      (i) Local recurrence
      (ii) Painful metastases
      (iii) Pathological fractures
   c. Medical
      (i) Anti-oestrogen/progesterone agents depending on receptor
          status
      (ii) Chemotherapy

12. Lymphatics and thymus

CAUSES OF LYMPH NODE ENLARGEMENT

1. Infections
    (i) Local enlargement, e.g. jugulodigastric node of tonsillitis
    (ii) General enlargement, e.g. mononucleosis, AIDS
2. Malignancy
    (i) Local enlargement, e.g. axilla in breast cancer
    (ii) General enlargement, e.g. lymphatic leukaemia, Hodgkin's

Always examine:
(i) Regional lymph nodes
(ii) Other nodes
(iii) Liver and spleen

HODGKIN'S DISEASE

Staging
I Single lymph node group involved, single extralymphatic organ or site involved
II Two or more node groups involved on same side of the diaphragm/localized involvement of extralymphatic organ and lymph nodes on same side of the diaphragm
III Lymph nodes on both sides of the diaphragm involved
IV Disseminated disease
    a. No systemic symptoms
    b. Systemic symptoms
        (i) Fever
        (ii) Weight loss
        (iii) Night sweats

Histological types
1. Lymphocyte dominant – favourable prognosis
2. Nodular sclerosing – favourable prognosis
3. Mixed cellularity – intermediate prognosis
4. Lymphocyte depleted – poor prognosis

Investigations
1. Chest X-ray, e.g. hilar nodes
2. Bone marrow biopsy
3. CAT scan – chest and/abdomen
4. Lymphangiogram and gallium scan
5. Staging laparotomy

Surgical procedures
1. Biopsy of presenting mass
2. Staging laparotomy
   (i) Liver biopsy
   (ii) Splenectomy
   (iii) Biopsy of lymph nodes (all major abdominal groups)

Rationale for staging laparotomy
1. Prognosis depends on staging
2. Treatment depends on staging
3. Physical examination, laboratory studies, X-rays and scans all have significant insensitivity
4. Surgical staging upgrades the clinical staging in approx. 30% and downstages it in 15% (total of 40% change)

Indications for staging
Depend to some extent on local policy. In general:
1. Any suspicion of abdominal involvement
2. Stage Ib/IIb patients with lymphocyte depleted or mixed cellular type of tumour
No indication for staging laparotomy: e.g. high cervical node involvement, lymphocyte predominant histology, and no evidence of mediastinal involvement, since it is very unusual for such patients to have abdominal disease

Principles of treatment
Stages:

I
II } Radiation therapy

IIIa
IIIb } Chemotherapy
IV

THYMUS

Myasthenia gravis – relationship to thymus
 (i) 15% of patients with myasthenia gravis have a thymoma
 (ii) Thymectomy is especially effective in young women with a short history and no thymoma

(iii) 40% of thymomas are malignant and surgery has better results than radiation therapy

(iv) Thymectomy may lower corticosteroid dose

LYMPHOEDEMA

Causes
1. Congenital
2. Following surgery, e.g. lymph node dissection
3. Malignant disease
4. Radiation therapy
5. Elephantiasis (filariasis)

Complications
1. Cellulitis
2. Lymphangitis
3. Lymphangiosarcoma (esp. following mastectomy and long-standing lymphoedema)

Treatment
1. Compression stockings
2. Avoid infections
3. Surgery – rarely indicated
   (i) Excision of subcutaneous tissue
   (ii) Lymphaticovenous anastomosis

13. Chest and lungs

CHEST INJURIES (BLUNT/PENETRATING)

Complications
1. Ribs: multiple fractures may cause flail chest
2. Pleura, lungs, bronchi:
   (i) Haemo-/haemopneumothorax
   (ii) Surgical emphysema
   (iii) Lung contusion
3. Heart
   (i) Cardiac tamponade
   (ii) Cardiac rupture
   (iii) Ruptured papillary muscle
   (iv) Ruptured valve
   (v) Lacerated coronary artery
4. Large vessels: haemothorax (see 'Rupture of aorta')
5. Oesophagus: mediastinitis
6. Diaphragm:
   (i) Herniation of viscera
   (ii) Injury to intra-abdominal organs

Principles of treatment
1. Airway: intubate – tracheostomy – positive pressure ventilation
2. Shock: blood and intravenous fluid
3. Chest drainage: of blood/air
4. Empty stomach to prevent aspiration
5. Thoracotomy
   (i) Haemorrhage which does not stop spontaneously.
   (ii) Bronchial disruption.
   (iii) Major vessel injury/tamponade

PNEUMOTHORAX

Causes
1. Spontaneous, e.g. ruptured bulla
2. Traumatic, e.g. sucking chest wound

3. Iatrogenic, e.g. pleural tap, lung biopsy, CVP line insertion, positive pressure ventilation

Signs of tension pneumothorax
1. Increasing dyspnoea and cyanosis
2. Inequality of breast sounds
3. Increasing displacement of mediastinum
4. Increasing peripheral venous congestion
5. Decreasing chest compliance during ventilation

CARDIAC TAMPONADE

Diagnosis
1. Think of possibility
2. Rising pulse rate
3. Falling blood pressure
4. Rising JVP
5. Diminished heart sounds
6. Pulsus paradoxus
7. Increasing cardiac outline on chest X-ray
8. Ultrasound
9. Emergency pericardiocentesis

LUNG ABSCESS

Causes
1. Tumour
    (i) Distal to airway obstruction
    (ii) Necrosis of tumour
2. Pneumonia
    (i) Especially staphylococcal
    (ii) TB
    (iii) Actinomycosis
3. Inhalation
    (i) Peanuts (children)
    (ii) Teeth
    (iii) Vomit, pus
    (iv) Food – achalasia/pharyngeal pouch, debilitated patient
4. Embolic
    (i) Septicaemic–SBE, intravenous drug addicts
    (ii) Infected pulmonary infarction
5. Infected lung cysts
6. Penetrating trauma
7. Subphrenic abscess – e.g. amoebic
8. Immunosuppression and general debility especially fungal and parasitic

Complications of lung abscess
1. Empyema
2. Pyopneumothorax
3. Cerebral abscess
4. Haemorrhage
5. Weight loss, anaemia

Treatment of lung abscess
1. Exclude bronchial obstruction
2. Dependent drainage
3. Antibiotics
4. Surgical drainage – open/percutaneous

EMPYEMA

Causes of empyema
1. Lung disease
   (i) Pneumonia
   (ii) TB
   (iii) Carcinoma
   (iv) Bronchiectasis
   (v) Postoperative
2. Ruptured oesophagus
3. Subphrenic spread
4. Septicaemia
5. Penetrating chest wound

Treatment of empyema
1. Acute
   (i) Thoracentesis and antibiotics
   (ii) Closed chest tube drainage if pus cannot be adequately aspirated via thoracentesis
2. Chronic
   (i) Open thoracotomy
   (ii) Decortication later if lung fails to expand

LUNG TUMOUR

Benign
1. Adenoma (carcinoid, cylindroma)
2. Hamartoma
3. Miscellaneous

Malignant – primary
1. Undifferentiated small cell (oat cell)
2. Squamous cell

3. Undifferentiated large cell
4. Adenocarcinoma
5. Alveolar bronchiolar cell carcinoma

Malignant – secondary
1. Breast
2. Kidney
3. Thyroid
4. Testis
5. Adrenal
6. Choriocarcinoma
7. Sarcoma, esp. bone
8. Melanoma

BRONCHIAL CARCINOMA

Effects
1. Bronchial obstruction
   (i) Collapse
   (ii) Recurrent pneumonia
   (iii) Abscess
   (iv) Empyema
2. Pleural involvement
   (i) Pain
   (ii) Effusion
   (iii) Pneumothorax
3. Neurological involvement
   (i) Brachial plexus: arm pain
   (ii) Sympathetic chain: Horner's syndrome
   (iii) Recurrent nerve: hoarseness
   (iv) Phrenic nerve: elevated diaphragm
4. Heart and pericardium
   (i) Pericardial effusion
   (ii) Atrial fibrillation
5. Blood vessels: SVC syndrome
6. Oesophagus: fistula
7. Lymphatics:
   (i) Chylothorax
   (ii) Lymphadenopathy
8. Blood spread
   (i) Bone: fractures
   (ii) Brain: epilepsy.
   (iii) Liver: jaundice
   (iv) Adrenals: adrenal cortical failure
9. Transcoelomic spread: pleural seedlings

Associated findings in bronchial carcinoma
1. Clubbing

2. Weight loss
3. Anaemia
4. Neuropathies
    (i) Peripheral
    (ii) Myelopathy
    (iii) Cerebellar degeneration
    (iv) Dementia
5. Myopathy
6. ACTH, PTH, ADH secretion, etc.

Pancoast's syndrome
1. Apical shadow on X-ray
2. Rib erosion
3. Horner's syndrome
4. Lower brachial plexus lesion

Investigation of bronchial carcinoma
1. Chest X-ray
2. Cytology of sputum or pleural fluid
3. Needle aspiration of lesion under X-ray or CT guidance
4. Brush biopsy
5. Bronchoscopy. May reveal:
    (i) Vocal cord paresis
    (ii) Tracheal compression
    (iii) Widening and loss of mobility carina
    (iv) In 75% cases the tumour is visible
6. CT scan – great advance in staging disease
7. Mediastinoscopy
8. Oesophagoscopy/barium swallow
9. Bone scan – if skeletal symptoms present

Treatment of bronchial carcinoma
1. Resectable lesions should be resected. Postoperative radiation can be given if nodes positive – controversial results
2. Radiation for unresectable lesions and complications (oat cell is most sensitive)
    (i) Reduces haemoptysis
    (ii) Reduces bone pain
    (iii) Relieves SVC obstruction
    (iv) May relieve cough and dyspnoea
3. Chemotherapy – generally in conjunction with radiation

CAUSES OF PLEURAL EFFUSION
1. Serous – transudates
    (i) Heart failure
    (ii) Liver failure

(iii) Nephrotic syndrome
2. Serous – exudates
   (i) Pneumonia
   (ii) Tumour
   (iii) Infarction (PE)
   (iv) Collagen disease
   (v) Subphrenic abscess
3. Purulent – see empyema
4. Haemorrhagic
   (i) Trauma
   (ii) Embolus
   (iii) Tumour
5. Chylous
   (i) Trauma
   (ii) Tumour
   (iii) Filariasis

ABNORMAL MEDIASTINAL MASS ON CHEST X-RAY

1. Superior mediastinum
   (i) Thyroid
   (ii) Aortic aneurysm
   (iii) Parathyroid adenoma – very rarely large enough
2. Anterior mediastinum
   (i) Thymoma
   (ii) Dermoid cysts and teratomas
   (iii) Hodgkin's, lymphosarcoma
   (iv) Pleuropericardial cyst
3. Middle mediastinum
   (i) Hilar lymph nodes
   (ii) Bronchogenic cysts
4. Posterior mediastinum
   (i) Achalasia of the cardia
   (ii) Hiatus hernia
   (iii) Neurofibroma

COMPLICATIONS OF TRACHEOSTOMY

1. At operation
   (i) Cardiac arrhythmia and arrest
   (ii) Haemorrhage
   (iii) Placing the incision too low in the trachea (predisposes to tracheo-innominate artery fistula)
   (iv) Injury to adjacent structures
2. Early postoperative
   (i) Displacement or obstruction of the tube
   (ii) Aspiration

   (iii) Tracheobronchial infection
   (iv) Tracheo-innominate artery fistula
    (v) Tracheo-oesophageal fistula
3. Late postoperative
    (i) Persistent stoma
   (ii) Tracheal stenosis
  (iii) Tracheomalacia
   (iv) Granuloma

SUPERIOR VENA CAVA SYNDROME

1. Headache
2. Confusion
3. Discomfort on bending over
4. Facial swelling, esp. eyelids
5. Distended veins in upper part of body
6. Hoarseness/dyspnoea form vocal cord swelling
7. Cerebral oedema
8. Intracranial thrombosis
9. Death

14. Vascular

PULSES TO BE ROUTINELY EXAMINED AND RECORDED

1. Lower limb
   (i) Aorta
   (ii) Femoral
   (iii) Popliteal
   (iv) Dorsalis pedis
   (v) Posterior tibial
2. Upper limb
   (i) Brachial
   (ii) Radial
   (iii) Ulnar
3. Neck: carotid

ARTERIAL OCCLUSION

Causes of arterial occlusion
1. In lumen
   (i) Thrombosis
      a. On an ulcerated plaque
      b. Hypercoagulable state, e.g. polycythaemia
   (ii) Embolus
      Sites – tend to lodge at vessel bifurcations, where diameter narrows abruptly
      a. Lower limb   70%
      b. Brain   20–25%
      c. Visceral arteries   5–10%
      Sources
      a. Heart 90%
         (i) Atrial fibrillation
         (ii) Mitral stenosis
         (iii) Post myocardial infarction (mural thrombus)
         (iv) Bacterial endocarditis
         (v) Myxoma
         (vi) Paradoxical (rare)

b. Elsewhere 10%
  (i) Arterio-arterial emboli
  (ii) Blue toe syndrome (aorta)
  (iii) Transient ischaemic attack (carotid)
  (iv) Raynaud's phenomenon (subclavian)
(iii) Atherosclerosis
  a. Aorto-iliac can present with Leriche's syndrome
    (i) Impotence
    (ii) Claudication – thigh, calf, and buttock
    (iii) Gangrene absent
  b. Femoro-popliteal occlusion – especially associated with cigarette smoking
  c. Tibio peroneal occlusion – especially associated with diabetics

2. In wall
  (i) Spasm: Raynaud's trauma
  (ii) Trauma
    a. Intimal flap, e.g. iatrogenic
    b. Transection

3. Outside vessel
  (i) Bone, e.g. supracondylar elbow fracture, knee dislocation
  (ii) Haematoma
  (iii) Plaster cast

Chronic ischaemia: clinical features

1. Claudication
  (i) Buttock pain – aorto-iliac disease
  (ii) Thigh pain – common femoral disease
  (iii) Calf pain – superficial femoral occlusion
  (iv) Ankle/foot pain – tibial artery occlusion, esp. diabetics
2. Rest pain: a symptom of severe ischaemia, and generally implies impending gangrene
3. Ulcer, gangrene (wet/dry), slow wound healing
4. Decreased, or loss of, pulses at rest or on exercise. Use of Doppler adds to routine examination by providing pressure measurement
   Ankle/arm pressure ratio can be calculated. Diabetics may have a falsely high ratio due to vessel rigidity.
  (i) Normal 1.0 or greater
  (ii) Claudication, often 0.5–1.0
  (iii) Severe ischaemia, less than 0.5
5. Loss of hair, brittle opaque nails, muscle atrophy, susceptibility to cold
6. Pallor of limb and worsening of pain on elevation
7. Dependent rubor (Bueger's sign) and improvement of pain in dependent position
8. Slow capillary return
9. Prolonged venous filling time (normal 10–15 seconds)

Acute arterial occlusion: clinical features ('Six Ps')
1. Pain. In a small number of patients the limb becomes numb immediately, and no pain is felt
2. Paralysis
3. Paraesthesia
4. Pulseless
5. Pallor
6. Perishing with cold

The presence of paraesthesia and paralysis signify nerve ischaemia. Gangrene can be set in within 6 hours unless circulation is restored

Treatment of chronic ischaemia
Intermittent claudication

Non-surgical
Only 5% patients progress to gangrene. Increased collateral circulation develops with time and symptoms often improve. Most patients succumb to stroke/MI
1. Patient education
   (i) Weight reduction
   (ii) Stop smoking
   (iii) Exercise programme
   (iv) Meticulous foot care; 40% of patients who undergo amputation give a history of trivial injury as the initiating event leading to the amputation
   (v) Heal raise
2. Control of diabetes and hypertension
3. Low dose aspirin

Surgery
For incapacitating symptoms in otherwise suitable patients. Operations are based on arteriographic findings and the general condition of the patient
1. Transluminal angioplasty (Gruntzig)
   (i) For short segmental areas of stenosis or occlusion
   (ii) 10% complication rate of vessel perforation or early occlusion
   (iii) Can be repeated
   (iv) Less invasive than open operation
   (v) Requires close cooperation between surgeon and radiologist
   (vi) Suitable for the following arteries:
      a. Coronary
      b. Mesenteric
      c. Renal
      d. Peripheral
2. Endarterectomy. Suitable for local areas of disease
   (i) Carotid

(ii) Profundaplasty
3. Bypass procedures
  (i) Aorto-iliac. Almost 100% patency rate
  (ii) Femoro-popliteal
    a. In situ saphenous vein – success depends on the adequacy of run-off vessels, e.g. 3 vessels better than 1 vessel
    b. Synthetic graft, e.g. Gortex, if vein unsuitable
  (iii) Extra anatomic
    a. Femoro-femoral, for unilateral iliac occlusion
    b. Axillo-femoral, for aorto-iliac occlusion in a patient who is considered too fragile to undergo aorto-iliac surgery
4. Sympathectomy
  (i) Used in some patients with unreconstructable situations
  (ii) Increases blood flow to the skin, but not to muscle
  (iii) May diminish pain
  (iv) May limit the extent of amputation
  (v) No way of predicting who will benefit
5. Amputation
  (i) Transmetatarsal
  (ii) Below knee
  (iii) Above knee
An arteriogram should always be strongly considered prior to amputation since arterial procedures may result in a lower level amputation or even limb salvage. Since patient who come to amputation are manifesting a local symptom of a generalized disease, the mortality and major complication rate is very high, e.g. stroke/MI

Treatment of acute arterial occlusion
Aim is to treat prior to onset of permanent muscle or nerve damage
1. Embolism
  (i) Heparinize to prevent propagation of thrombus
  (ii) Embolectomy (Fogarty catheter). Must remove the propagated thrombus. Operative arteriogram often required
  (iii) Fasciotomy may be needed
  (iv) Continue anticoagulation to protect from further emboli
2. Acute arterial thrombosis
  (i) Embolectomy
  (ii) Correction of circulatory problem, e.g. bypass

VASCULAR INJURY

Pathology
1. Spasm – must not be confused with contusion
2. Thrombosis
3. Division
4. Intimal tear

5. Aneurysm
6. Arteriovenous fistula

Diagnosis
1. Arterial injury may be present even in the presence of a normal pulse distal to the injury (20%)
2. There may be brisk bleeding or a haematoma
3. Bruit may be present
4. Arteriogram may be needed to make diagnosis especially in blunt trauma

THE DIABETIC FOOT

1. Very prone to infection. Often follows trivial trauma and can result in necrotizing infections of the interdigital space which rapidly spread proximally
2. Diabetic neuropathy. Causes painless ulcers, which then are an entry site for infection
3. Arterial occlusive disease involving the popliteal artery and its branches down to pedal arches
4. Patients with foot pain from diabetic neuropathy do not obtain relief with dependency, distinguishing them from patients with pain on the basis of atherosclerosis

ANEURYSMS

Aetiology
1. Congenital, e.g. berry aneurysm
2. Traumatic, e.g. false aneurysm
3. Inflammatory, e.g. SBE
4. Degenerative, e.g. atheromatous

Complications
1. Rupture, esp. aortic
2. Thrombosis ⎤ esp. peripheral – popliteal, femoral, carotid
3. Embolism ⎦
4. Infection, esp. salmonella
5. Pressure, e.g. dysphagia from thoracic aortic aneurysm

Abdominal aortic aneurysms
1. For aneurysms 5 cm in diameter or larger, 20% chance of rupture per year. Size may best be measured by ultrasound
2. While most ruptures are preceded by some warning symptoms some are not, and therefore resection is advised when the diagnosis is made. Emergency mortality rate is ten times higher

3. Onset of symptoms implies impending rupture, and need for urgent operation
   (i) Low back pain/sciatica
   (ii) Renal colic type pain
   (iii) Any acute abdominal condition
4. Failure to palpate the abdomen carefully and consider the diagnosis is the chief cause for delay in treatment
5. Complications of aneurysm resection
   (i) Renal failure
   (ii) Declamping shock
   (iii) Peripheral embolization
   (iv) Ischaemic necrosis of the colon
   (v) Myocardial infarction
   (vi) Graft infection
   (vii) Graft enteric fitulae
   (viii) False aneurysms at suture line

Popliteal artery aneurysm
1. 25% are bilateral
2. Thrombosis or embolism can complicate them without warning
3. Urgent elective resection as soon as diagnosis is made

ARTERIOVENOUS FISTULA

1. Signs
   (i) Thrill
   (ii) Dilated pulsating veins
   (iii) Continuous murmur
2. Complications
   (i) Skin ulceration
   (ii) Limb hypertrophy (children)
   (iii) Heart failure (rare)
   (iv) SBE (rare)

CAUSES OF SURGICALLY CORRECTABLE HYPERTENSION

1. Unilateral renal disease, e.g. renal artery stenosis
2. Coarctation of the aorta
3. Phaeochromocytoma
4. Conn's syndrome
5. Cushing's syndrome

RAYNAUD'S PHENOMENON

Pallor – cyanosis – rubor. Precipitated by cold/emotion

Causes

Primary Raynaud's
No serious underlying cause

Secondary Raynaud's
1. Buerger's disease
2. Scleroderma
3. Cervical ribs
4. Vibrating tools
5. SLE
6. Blood disorders, e.g. cryoglobulinaemia

Raynaud's may precede signs of the above diseases by up to 3–5 years. Therefore primary Raynaud's is a tentative diagnosis.

Features
1. Unilateral cases imply a mechanical cause
2. About 15% have leg involvement
3. Focal ulcers and paronychia can develop
4. Arteriogram shows spasm in response to cold

Treatment
1. Avoid cold – most cases are mild and this suffices
2. Oral methyldopa has had some success
3. Intra-arterial reserpine
4. Sympathectomy – severe cases only, can be followed by relapse

DISSECTING ANEURYSMS
1. Hypertension with cystic medial necrosis is most important predisposing factor (also Marfan's syndrome)
2. 60 – 70% originate in aorta just distal to the aortic valve; 25% originate just distal to left subclavian take-off
3. Usually presents with sudden excruciating chest pain
4. Symptoms arise from complications
   (i) Rupture
      a. Pericardium – tamponade
      b. Mediastinum – shock
      c. Peritoneum – shock
   (ii) Occlusion of vessels

a. Coronary	Myocardial infarction
b. Head	Stroke
c. Intercostals	Spinal cord infarction
d. Renals	Anuria
e. Mesenteric	Bowel infarction
f. Iliacs	Limb ischaemia

Marfan, - AO - CT dis
arachnodactyly, high-arched palate, arm span > height
lens dislocation, aortic incompetence.

(iii) Aortic incompetence
5. Treatment
    (i) Early emergency aortography/CT
    (ii) Hypotensive therapy (e.g. nitroprusside and propranolol)
    (iii) Surgical correction

TRAUMATIC RUPTURE OF THORACIC AORTA

1. Commonly follows decelerating type of closed chest injury
2. Rupture occurs just distal to origin of left subclavian artery at site of ligamentum arteriosum
3. May be minimal clinical findings
    (i) Discrepancy between upper and lower limb pulse pressures
    (ii) Widened thoracic knob on chest X-ray
4. Requires urgent repair

SUPERIOR VENA CAVA OBSTRUCTION

Causes
1. Malignancy 90%
    (i) Lung
    (ii) Lymphoma
    (iii) Breast
2. Non-malignant cause
    Thoracic aneurysm

Clinical features
1. Headache
2. Eyelid swelling
3. Neck enlargement
4. Facial swelling
5. Cerebral oedema – severe cases

Treatment
1. Radiation/chemotherapy depending on cause
2. Surgical bypass really indicated

VARICOSE VEINS

Clinical Features
1. Phlebitis
2. Brawny oedema – generally imples perforator incompetence
3. Ulceration
4. Dermatitis
    (i) Allergy to locally applied drugs
    (ii) Fungal infection

5. Pigmentation
6. Cramps
7. Haemorrhage
8. Marjolin's ulcer

Treatment
1. Patient education
   (i) Avoid prolonged standing
   (ii) Wear effective support stockings
2. Injection therapy, esp. for varicosities below the knee
3. Sapheno-femoral disconnection and stripping, with ligation of incompetent perforators (detected by Trendelenburg test)
   Varicose ulcer
   (i) If the ulcer is kept above the level of the heart it will heal
   (ii) Bed rest and elevation
   (iii) Systemic antibiotics if infected
   (iv) Small clean ulcers can be managed with firm support, e.g. paste boot
   (v) Treatment of varicose veins and perforators followed by excision of ulcer and skin grafting may be necessary

DIFFERENTIAL DIAGNOSIS OF LEG ULCERS

1. Venous stasis ulcers
2. Ischaemic ulcer
3. Neurotropic ulcer
4. Malignant ulcer
5. Ulcers complicating rheumatoid arthritis, ulcerative colitis, acholuric jaundice, sickle cell disease, collagen diseases
6. Dermatitis artefacta
7. Syphllis (gumma)

15. Oesophagus and diaphragm

CAUSES OF DYSPHAGIA

1. Oral and pharyngeal
    (i) Pharyngitis, e.g. monilia, postoperatively
    (ii) Retropharyngeal abscess
    (iii) Oral carcinoma
    (iv) Epiglottitis
    (v) Pharyngeal pouch
    (vi) Neuromuscular diseases
2. Oesophageal lesions
    a. Intraluminal: foreign bodies
    b. Intramural:
        (i) Trauma endoscopy
        (ii) Stricture acid/bile reflux
        (iii) Malignancy
        (iv) Achalasia
        (v) Plummer–Vinson syndrome
        (vi) Scleroderma
        (vii) Atresia
    c. Extraluminal
        (i) Goitre, esp. retrosternal
        (ii) Bronchial carcinoma
        (iii) Lymphadenopathy
3. General
    (i) Polio, syringomyelia
    (ii) Myasthenia
    (iii) Diphtheria

ACHALASIA OF THE CARDIA

Pathophysiology
1. Failure of the lower oesophageal sphincter to relax during swallowing
2. Absence of normal peristalsis in whole oesophagus
3. Degeneration of Auerbach's plexus seen in 2/3 cases

4. 7-fold increase in squamous cell cancer of the oesophagus

Clinical presentation
1. Intermittent dysphagia initially which becomes progressive
2. More difficulty with cold liquids initially
3. Pain is unusual except early in the disease
4. Paroxysmal nocturnal coughing and aspiration occur often
5. Barium swallow shows rat-tail deformity and frequently absent gastric air bubble
6. Treated by Heller's operation (cardiomyotomy) or pneumatic dilatation

ZENKER'S DIVERTICULUM

Pathophysiology
1. Pulsion diverticulum between thyro- and cricopharyngeus. The mouth of the diverticulum is above the superior oesophageal sphincter
2. Secondary to premature contraction of cricopharyngeus on swallowing

Clinical features
1. Dysphagia
2. Gurgling noises
3. Aspiration
4. Nocturnal coughing
5. Can be perforated during endoscopy
6. Malignancy is rare

Treatment
1. Resection of the diverticulum ± cricopharyngomyotomy
2. Suspension of diverticulum + cricopharyngomyotomy

DIAPHRAGMATIC HERNIA

Classification
1. Hiatus hernia
   a. Sliding, 90%. Hernia has a partial parietal peritoneal sac, and the gastro-oesophageal junction lies in the chest
   b. Rolling, 10% (paraoesophageal). The gastro-oesophageal junction lies in the normal position. May ultimately lead to an upside-down stomach. A pure paraoesophageal hernia is rare
2. Anterior hernia of Morgagni
3. Posterolaterall hernia of Bochdalek
4. Post-traumatic

Complications
1. Sliding hiatus hernia
   There is an association with reflux osophagitis, however reflux
   can occur independently of the presence of a sliding hernia
2. Rolling/paraoesophageal hiatus hernia
   (i) Haemorrhage
   (ii) Obstruction
   (iii) Incarceration
   (iv) Volvulus — _to vrtng ... dostruct & con of blood spply_
   (v) Intrathoracic gastric dilatation
3. Bochdalek — _Postero-lateral_
   Cause of acute respiratory distress in the newborn
4. Morgagni
   Herniation of bowel, etc. Most are asymptomatic

REFLUX OESOPHAGITIS

Normal physiology
1. High pressure zone in region of the cardia
   (i) No histological sphincter in humans, but intrinsic oesophageal
       muscle is responsive to hormones, e.g. gastrin
   (ii) Intra-abdominal segment of oesophagus is at positive
       pressure with respect to intrathoracic portion
2. Other, probably less important factors:
   (i) Acute gastro–oesophageal angle forming flap valve
       mechanism
   (ii) Pinchcock effect of right crus of diaphragm
   (iii) Mucosal folds

Symptoms
1. Heartburn
2. Regurgitation
3. Dysphagia
4. Bleeding
5. Choking
6. Coughing

Differential diagnosis
1. Angina pectoris
2. Biliary disease
3. Diverticulitis
4. Peptic ulcer

Investigations
1. Endoscopy. Symptoms and degree of inflammation not
   necessarily correlated. Provides means of biopsy
2. Manometry. Measures lower sphincter pressure

3. 24-hour, pH monitoring of distal oesophageal
4. Acid clearing test
5. Acid perfusion test of Bernstein
6. Radioactive scanning, e.g. ^{99m}Tc
7. Barium swallow

Causes of reflux oesophagitis
1. Reflux
2. Caustic/acid ingestion
3. Infection, e.g. candida, especially diabetics, steroids
4. Prolonged vomiting
5. Nasogastric tube

Complications
1. Bleeding
2. Stricture
3. Shortening of oesophagitis
4. Oesophageal ulcer perforation
5. Motility disorders
6. Barrett oesophagus. (Columnar epithelium replaces normal squamous epithelium for a variable distance up the oeso-phagus)

Treatment of reflux oesophagitis
1. Elevate head of bed
2. Avoid lying or stooping after meals
3. Avoid constricting clothing
4. Antacids, histamine receptor antagonists, metoclopramide
5. Surgery

Indications for surgery
Aim of operation is to restore competence to the lower oeso-phageal sphincter. A variety of operations exist (Nissen, Belsey, etc.)
1. Failed medical treatment
2. Bleeding
3. Stricture
4. Severe ulceration
5. Paraoesophageal hernia

RUPTURED OESOPHAGUS

Causes
1. Endoscopy – most common cause and mostly cervical
2. Forceful vomiting (Boerhaave syndrome). Lower oesophagus
3. Sharp ingested foreign body
4. Postoperative, e.g. vagotomy, hiatus hernia repair

5. External trauma
6. Neoplasm

Clinical features
1. A highly lethal condition
2. Successful treatment depends on early diagnosis
3. Site of perforation and interval between perforation and diagnosis influence findings
4. Pain, fever, dysphagia – most frequent early complaints

Sites of perforation
1. Cervical perforation
   (i) Cervical tenderness
   (ii) Crepitation
   (iii) Supraclavicular abscess – late
2. Thoracic perforation
   (i) Crunching precordial sounds – mediastinal emphysema
   (ii) Mediastinitis
   (iii) Pleural effusion – hydropneumothorax
   (iv) Empyema
3. Infradiaphragmatic – generalized peritonitis

Treatment
1. Cervical
   (i) Drainage – not always necessary
   (ii) Antibiotics
2. All others
   (i) Close perforation (in early cases)
   (ii) Adequate drainage
   (iii) Antibiotics
   (iv) Maintain nutrition

OESOPHAGEAL CANCER

Risk factors
1. Alcoholism, tobacco
2. Plummer–Vinson syndrome
3. Corrosive oesophagitis
4. Males >50 years
5. Achalasia
6. Geographical, e.g. South Africa
7. Barrett oesophagus

Pathology of oesophageal carcinoma

Distribution	Frequency	Cell type
Cervical	10%	Squamous
Upper third	20%	Squamous
Middle third	20%	Squamous
Lower third	50%	Adenocarcinoma 90%

Clinical features
1. Progressive dysphagia
2. Weight loss
3. Aspiration pneumonia

Diagnosis
1. History
2. Endoscopy and biopsy – establishes histology and limits of lesion
3. Barium swallow
4. Cytology by washing/abrasion technique (used for screening in China)
5. CT scanning helps to determine mediastinal involvement
6. Bronchoscopy may be needed to exclude bronchial involvement in upper lesions

Treatment
1. One-third of patients present in an advanced stage of disease, but are very symptomatic and require palliation
2. Radiation is more effective for squamous lesions, however there is a high local recurrence rate/complication rate (stricture, fistula etc.)
3. Surgery provides most rapid palliation, and shortest treatment time, so that if a lesion is resectable, surgery should be the prime choice in an otherwise suitable patient. Most operations involve resection of the oesophagus and mobilization of the stomach to make up the defect
4. For very advanced disease, the use of indwelling tubes to allow swallowing is only partially successful. Recently endoscopic laser resection of tumours has been shown to provide good palliation
5. Early detection of lesions (Hunan, China) has been shown to improve the cure rate greatly

BARRETT OESOPHAGUS

In response to chronic reflux, squamous cell lining of the oesophagus is replaced by columnar (non-acid secreting) mucosa. Ulceration and stricture can occur. There is an increased incidence of malignancy.

Exact risk unknown. Improvement may be seen following correction of reflux in some cases

RUPTURE OF THE DIAPHRAGM

1. Usually follows blunt trauma
2. More commonly on the left
3. Commonly part of a more severe injury
4. Commonly missed and presents years later with an abnormal chest X-ray
5. Inspection of the diaphragm should be included in exploratory laparotomy following trauma

16. Stomach and duodenum

PEPTIC ULCER DISEASE

Mucosal defect arising in or adjacent to acid secreting epithelium

Duodenal ulcer group
Tend to have high normal/excess acid secretion
1. Duodenal ulcers – 1st portion usually
2. Pyloric canal ulcer
3. Combined gastric and duodenal ulcer
4. Stomal ulcer
5. Zollinger–Ellison syndrome
6. Antral G cell hyperplasia

Gastric ulcer group
Tend to have normal or low acid output
Ulcers occur on the lesser curve at the junction of antral and fundic mucosa

Clinical features
1. Interval dyspepsia
2. Pain bears some relationship to food – mostly relieved
3. Pain awakens patient at night
4. May present with complication of peptic ulcer disease and no antecedent history
5. Differentiation of anatomical site on basis of history is unreliable

Investigation
1. Barium meal
2. Endoscopy
3. Acid secretion studies. May be used prior to deciding on type of operation
4. Gastrin assay, if Z-E syndrome or G cell hyperplasia are being considered
5. Exclude co-existing disease

Management of duodenal ulcer group

Medical
1. Eat small amounts frequently

2. Avoid stress
3. Avoid ulcerogenic drugs
4. Stop smoking
5. H_2 receptor antagonists or omeprazole
6. Antacids

Surgical
1. Elective surgery for intractable cases
2. Emergency surgery for complications

Elective surgery
Aim is to reduce acid secretion within minimum morbidity, mortality, and lowest recurrent ulcer rate
1. Vagotomy. Abolishes neural stimulation of parietal cells, and reduces parietal cell response to stimuli, e.g. gastrin
   (i) Truncal vagotomy + drainage procedure
   (ii) Selective vagotomy + drainage procedure. Preserves vagal innervation of liver and small bowel. Results in less diarrhoea
   (iii) Highly selective vagotomy. Denervates parietal cell mass and preserves innervation of the pylorus. Drainage procedure not required. No diarrhoea
2. Antrectomy. Reduces the gastrin stimulus to the parietal cell

Results of surgery
1. Patents with intractable symptoms who spontaneously request surgery generally have the best result
2. Type of operation is best tailored to the patient and findings at surgery
   a. Thin patient – avoid gastrectomy
   b. Heavily scarred duodenum – may make gastrectomy hazardous
3. Highly selective vagotomy is accompanied by the lowest morbidity and side-effects and has emerged as ideal operation for many patients. Recurrences following this operation can usually be managed with H_2 receptor antagonists, or more extensive surgery

Procedure	20-year recurrence rate (%)
Truncal/selective vagotomy + drainage	5–25
Vagotomy and antrectomy	1
Partial gastrectomy	5
Highly selective vagotomy	5–10

Management of gastric ulcer group

Medical
1. Stop smoking

2. Antacids
3. Sulphated glycoproteins, e.g. sucralfate

Surgical
1. Elective for intractable cases
2. Emergency for complications

Indications for surgery of gastric ulcer
1. Any question of malignancy
2. Very large ulcers – increased risk of bleeding or perforation
3. Failure to diminish in size by 50% after 3 weeks of medical treatment
4. Pyloric channel ulcer – respond poorly to medical management
5. If associated with duodenal lulcer – tend to recur
6. Recurrent ulcer

Operations for gastric ulcer
Unlike the sitaution in the duodenum where an ulcer is for practical purposes always benign, gastric ulcers may be malignant. Biopsy carries a false negative rate of about 5%, and this must be remembered in choosing the type of operation for gastric ulcer
1. Partial gastrectomy including the ulcer results in a low recurrence rate (Billroth I)
2. High lying lesser curve ulcers pose a special problem since they may be close to the gastro-oesophageal junction and resection of this area carries much morbidity. Choices include local resection or leaving the ulcer in place in conjunction with vagotomy and drainage
3. More distal ulcers, in particular involving the pyloric channel, should be managed as duodenal ulcers

Specific complications of gastrectomy
a. Early complications
   1. Haemorrhage – suture line, ruptured spleen, coagulation defect
   2. Pancreatitis
   3. Duodenal stump leak
   4. Afferent loop obstruction (may occur late) – presents like pancreatitis with elevated amylase. Nasogastric aspirate is bile-free. Requires urgent surgery to prevent duodenal rupture
   5. Efferent loop obstruction
   6. Loop intussusception
   7. Anastromotic leak
   8. Subphrenic abscess
   9. Oesophageal rupture during vagotomy
   10. Gastro-ileostomy – failure to correctly identify the ligament of Treitz. Causes profound weight loss.

b. Later complications
   1. Dumping syndrome, 5–10% incidence
      a. Early: occurs within 10 minutes of eating and lasts 40–60 minutes. Caused by premature entry of hypertonic fluid into the duodenum
      b. Late: occurs about 2 hours after eating. Caused by hypoglycaemia secondary to excess insulin release
      c. Clinical features include:
         (i) Weakness, sweating, pallor
         (ii) Epigastric discomfort, and borborygmi
         (iii) Palpitations
         (iv) Diarrhoea
   2. Small capacity syndrome. Follows extensive resections
   3. Bilious vomiting
   4. Malabsorption
      (i) Iron deficiency anaemia
      (ii) Impaired B_{12} absorption
      (iii) Calcium, esp. with steatorrhoea
   5. Steatorrhoea
      (i) More common after Billroth II
      (ii) Gastric emptying and pancreatico-biliary secretions out of phase
      (iii) Colonization of afferent loop with bile salt splitting bacteria
   6. Diarrhoea
      (i) May follow vagotomy
      (ii) Cathartic effect of bile salts
      (iii) Steatorrhoea
      (iv) Bacterial overgrowth
   7. Recurrent ulcer or stomal ulcer
      a. Causes
         (i) Inadequate gastric resection or incomplete vagotomy
         (ii) Retained antrum at tip of afferent loop
         (iii) Z-E syndrome
      b. Complications
         (i) Haemorrhage
         (ii) Perforation
         (iii) Gastrojejunocolic fistula – best seen on barium enema
   8. Stomal obstruction, bezoar, citrus fruit
   9. Increased risk of carcinoma in the gastric remnant

Complications of peptic ulcer disease
1. Haemorrhage
2. Perforation
3. Pyloric obstruction

Management of complications

1. Haemorrhage
  (i) Replace blood volume using all necessary monitoring
  (ii) Endoscopy. A visible vessel in the bed of an ulcer implies a high risk of rebleeding. Yag laser has been used with success to stop bleeding
  (iii) Most cases stop spontaneously with combination of antacids and saline lavage
  (iv) In cases of persistent or recurrent bleeding emergency surgery may be necessary. Each case is a matter of judgement requiring close co-operation between physician and surgeon
  (v) Operation involves control of bleeding and anti-ulcer operation

2. Perforation
75% occur on anterior wall of lst portion of duodenum
  (i) Preoperative resuscitation
  (ii) Closure of perforation with omental patch
    a. In poor risk patients
    b. In patients with no antecedent history
    c. If treatment is delayed
  (iii) Addition of ulcer procedure to closure, e.g. highly selective vagotomy
    a. Prior ulcer history
    b. Good risk patient and no delay in treatment

3. Pyloric obstruction
  (i) Spasm – duodenitis – improves with intense medical therapy
  (ii) Scarring – chronic ulcer – requires definitive ulcer surgery
  (iii) Carcinoma – requires palliative resection

ACUTE GASTRIC MUCOSAL EROSIONS

Superficial to muscularis mucosa. Most occur in the fundus of stomach.

Causes
  1. Stress
    (i) Trauma
    (ii) Burns
    (iii) Operations
    (iv) Sepsis
  2. Alcohol
  3. Aspirin, phenylbutazone, indomethacin

Treatment
1. Prevention. Maintain gastric pH >5 (antacids/H$_2$ blockers)
2. For established bleeding
   (i) Maintain intravascular volume
   (ii) Antacids/H$_2$ blockers to stop acid secretion and raise pH
   (iii) Saline lavage to reduce fibrinolysins, and antral distension. Over 80% cases will cease bleeding with the above measures. If they fail, the following can be considered, bearing in mind one is generally dealing with a critically ill patient:
   (iv) Endoscopic coagulation – neodymium-Yag laser
   (v) Vasopressin infusion via left gastric artery
   (vi) Operation
       a. Highly selective vagotomy with oversew of erosions
       b. Oversew of bleeding erosions, vagotomy, pyloroplasty
       c. Vagotomy, gastrectomy
       d. Gastric devascularization
       e. Total gastrectomy – seldom if ever indicated

GASTRIC MALIGNANCY

Types
1. Adenocarcinoma – 95%
2. Lymphoma – 4%
3. Leiomyosarcomas – 1%

Predisposing factors for adenocarcinoma
1. Pernicious anaemia
2. Blood group A
3. Prior gastrectomy
4. Family history of gastric cancer

Clinical features
1. Anorexia and weight loss >95%
2. Pyloric obstruction
3. Haematemesis 5%
4. Dysphagia with proximal lesions
5. Pain – late
6. Palpable mass – 50%
7. Hepatomegaly
8. Peritoneal seedlings. May lead to:
   (i) Ascites
   (ii) Ovarian mass (Krukenberg's tumour)
   (iii) Mass in pelvic cul de sac (Bloomer's shelf)
9. Enlarged left supraclavicular lymph node (Virchow's node)
10. May present with perforation

Diagnosis
1. History, esp. unexplained weight loss
2. Endoscopy and biopsy
3. Barium meal
   (i) Space occupying mass
   (ii) Greater curve ulcer
   (iii) Rigidity of adjacent gastric wall
   (iv) Irregular or asymmetric crater
   (v) Mucosal folds do not radiate towards the ulcer
   (vi) Small thickened contracted stomach (linitis plastica)
   (vii) Fundic tumours are difficult to evaluate because of poor filling
   (viii) Gastric carcinoma can fulfil the radiological criteria for healing. Therefore biopsy is mandatory

Treatment
Requires a gastrectomy, the extent of which is dictated by the operative findings. In general total gastrectomy is avoided because of its attendant morbidity
1. Curative in a minority of patients, since lymph node involvement has occurred in 50% cases. In Japan screening has led to early diagnosis and increased cure rate
2. Palliative. Prevents bleeding, perforation, and obstruction

ACUTE GASTRIC DILATATION

Causes
1. Postoperative, e.g. cholecystectomy
2. Trauma, e.g. chest/abdomen
3. Patients on positive pressure ventilators
4. Plaster of Paris jacket application

Clinal features
1. Hiccoughs
2. Periodic regurgitation
3. Hypotension, oliguria, tachycardia
4. Managed by placing a nasogastric tube

MALLORY–WEISS SYNDROME

1. Massive haematemesis following forceful vomiting (alcoholism, pregnancy
2. Longitudinal mucosal tear at gastro-oesophageal junction
3. Most stop bleeding spontaneously
4. Sengstaken–Blakemore tube can be helpful
5. Operation is rarely required

GASTRIC VOLVULUS

1. May be mesentero-axial/organoaxial
2. Accompanied by nausea, vomiting, retching
3. Nasogastric tube will not pass into stomach
4. Emergency surgery required if spontaneous reduction does not occur rapidly

GASTROINTESTINAL HAEMORRHAGE

Causes

1. General bleeding disorders
2. Oesophagus
   (i) Varices
   (ii) Oesophagitis
   (iii) Mallory–Weiss syndrome
3. Stomach
   (i) Ulcer
   (ii) Erosions
   (iii) Tumours
4. Duodenum
   (i) Ulcer
   (ii) Ampullary tumour
   (iii) Haemobilia
5. Small intestine
   (i) Meckel's
   (ii) Tumour
6. Large bowel
   (i) Diverticulitis
   (ii) Carcinoma
   (iii) Inflammatory bowel disease
   (iv) Polyps
   (v) Haemorrhoids
7. Aortic aneurysms or prosthetic grafts may rupture into the oesophagus or duodenum
8. Vascular anomalies, e.g. haemangioma, hereditary telangiectasia

Most common causes of upper gastrointestinal haemorrhage
1. Peptic ulcers 50–65%
2. Erosions 30%
3. Varices 5%
For management see specific sections

Most common causes of lower gastrointestinal bleeding
1. Children
   (i) Meckel's diverticulum
   (ii) Polyps
   (iii) Ulcerative colitis

2. Adults
   (i) Haemorrhoids
   (ii) Vascular ectasia
       a. Occur in patients over 60 years
       b. Occur in right colon
       c. Small, <5 mm
       d. Identifiable only on angiography, not at operation
   (iii) Diverticulosis
   (iv) Polyps (benign/malignant)
   (v) Carcinoma
   (vi) Congenital arteriovenous malformations

Investigation of gastrointestinal bleeding

1. 4–6 hourly haematocrit levels
2. PTT, PT, platelet count
3. Endoscopy
4. ^{99m}Tc-labelled red cells. Scanning can be continued for up to 24 hours
5. Arteriography. Bleeding must be at the rate of 3–5 ml/minute
6. Emergency laparotomy. Occasional patients cannot be diagnosed by any of these tests or bleeding may be so rapid that immediate exploration is necessary to save the patient's life. In general however every effort should be made to have a diagnosis before surgery, as it is frequently difficult to identify a bleeding site at operation

17. Bowel tumours

POLYPS

Polyp is a term with no histopathological implications desribing a mass of tissue arising from mucosa that protrudes into the bowel lumen

Classification
1. Neoplastic
   a. Benign
      (i) Tubular adenoma
      (ii) Villous adenoma
      (iii) Tubulovillous
   b. Malignant
      Adenocarcinoma
2. Hamartomata – no malignant potential
   (i) Peutz–Jegher's syndrome
   (ii) Juvenile polyp
3. Inflammatory
   Pseudopolyposis in inflammatory bowel disease
4. Familial adenomatous polyposis coli
   a. Autosomal dominant
   b. Malignancy certain eventually

Clinical features

Adenomatous polyps
1. Most common colonic neoplasm
2. 70% are within reach of the sigmoidoscope
3. Malignant potential increased with polyp size (<1 cm in size, <1% malignant; 1–2 cm, 10% malignant)
4. May present with bleeding, prolapse, and rarely intussusception, but most commonly are asymptomatic
5. Colonoscopic polypectomy has simplified management

Villous adenoma
1. May present with blood or mucus in stool

2. May cause hypokalaemia
3. 80% occur in the rectosigmoid
4. 30% actively invasive. 30% have atypical cellularity
5. Hard areas within the polyp correlate well with malignancy
6. Non-invasive low lying lesions are locally resected per anus.
   Partial colectomy with primary anastomosis for higher lesions

Familial adenomatous polyposis coli
1. Autosomal dominant inheritance – screen all relatives
2. Colonic polyps appear around 13 years
3. 100% malignant potential
4. Bleeding often heralds malignant change which carries a poor
   prognosis
5. Treatment
   (i) Panproctocolectomy with permanent ileostomy
   (ii) Ileoanal pouch
   (iii) Ileorectal anastomosis
6. Associated later in life with:
   (i) Small bowel tumours, esp. duodenum (potentially malignant)
   (ii) Desmoid tumours of bowel mesentery. Ongoing surveillance
       required following colectomy

Gardner's syndrome
1. Autosomal dominant inheritance
2. Polyps appear later (30s), and may involve small bowel
3. Cancer occurs later and less frequently
4. Associated with:
   a. Osteomas, exostoses (mandible, skull, sinuses)
   b. Epidermoid or sebaceous cysts
   c. Desmoid tumours, esp. in abdominal incisions
   d. Postoperative mesenteric fibromatosis
5. Colectomy for colonic polyps

COLORECTAL CARCINOMA

Predisposing factors
1. Ulcerative colitis
2. Familial polyposis coli
3. Villous tumours
4. Gardner's syndrome
5. Adenomatous polyps
6. Family history of GI cancer

Sites
There has been a gradual shift proximally, so that fewer carcinomas
can be felt on rectal examination
1. 35% within reach of rigid sigmoidoscope

2. 35% in caecum and ascending colon
3. Approx. 5% have a second primary

Spread
1. Direct extension: through bowel wall into adjacent structures
2. Lymphatic spread. Mesenteric, and para-aortic nodes
3. Bloodstream: liver, lung, bone
4. Transcoelomic: cul-de-sac (Bloomer's shelf), omentum, ovaries (Kruckenberg)
5. Implantation at operation, e.g. anastomotic recurrence

Staging
Dukes' system has gained most widespread recognition

Stage	Depth	5-year survival (%)
A	Limited to muscularis mucosa	98
B1	Extends to muscularis propria	
B2	Extends through muscularis propria	78
C1	Involved nodes all removed (gross)	
C2	Involved nodes remain following resection	32
D	Distant metastasis	6

Clinical presentation
1. Change in bowel habit
   (i) Constipation
   (ii) Diarrhoea
   (iii) Decreased stool calibre
2. Rectal bleeding – gross/occult
3. Obstruction – esp. left side
4. Perforation – free or with abscess formation
5. Nagging pain, anaemia, weight loss – esp. right-sided lesions
6. Fistulization to stomach or bladder
7. General cachexia, ascites, jaundice

Investigation
1. Rectal examination
2. Rigid/flexible sigmoidoscopy
3. Colonoscopy
4. Barium studies
5. IVP/CT scanning sometimes indicated

Treatment of colorectal cancer

Preoperative
1. Bowel preparation for elective cases
2. Prophylactic antibiotics

Operation
Extent is guided by the operative findings, and the general condition of the patient
1. Right hemicolectomy – caecal, ascending, and hepatic flexure lesions
2. Transverse colectomy – mid transverse lesions
3. Left hemicolectomy – splenic flexure, descending lesions
4. Sigmoid colectomy – sigmoid lesions
5. Anterior resection – rectosigmoid lesions
6. Abdominoperineal resection – very low rectal lesions
7. Radiation/fulguration to treat low rectal tumours
8. Local excision/fulguration of tumour to prevent bleeding/obstruction in patients too sick to tolerate major operation
9. Patients presenting with obstruction may require a temporary colostomy as part of the operation if the bowel cannot be prepared before operation or is not suitable for on-table lavage

Resection of isolated hepatic metastases
Controversial, but being performed increasingly frequently

Role and timing of radiation therapy
Still not well defined
1. May decrease size of bulky lesions, enabling resection
2. May decrease local recurrence rate

Chemotherapy
1. Combination of 5-FU and radiation may reduce local recurrence following resection of transmural rectal carcinoma
2. 5-FU and leucovorin adjuvant therapy for patients with positive nodes following colectomy

Treatment of recurrent disease
1. Small bowel obstruction due to recurrent cancer may require exploration but results are often disappointing
2. Radiation may provide relief for perineal or bone pain
3. Some liver metastases may be worth resecting
4. Patients are at risk of developing further colon tumours – regular follow up colonoscopy is recommended to look for early disease or polyps

FACTORS PREDISPOSING TO ANASTOMOTIC LEAK
1. Poor surgical technique
   (i) Poorly placed sutures
   (ii) Sutures tied too tight
   (iii) Injury to tissues from rough handling

    (iv) Poor blood supply
    (v) Tension
2. Contamination
3. Surrounding infection
4. Low rectal anastomoses
5. Prior radiation (preop radiation does not impair healing if operation is carried out within about 6 weeks of completion)
6. Drain in contact with anastomosis

EARLY DETECTION OF COLON CANCER

1. Testing for occult blood
    (i) 25% carcinomas do not bleed enough to cause positive result
    (ii) 75% of adenomatous polyps do not bleed
    (iii) 60% of cancers detected by this test are Duke A/B c.f. 30% detected by other means
2. Routine sigmoidoscopy in patients over 40 years probably not cost-effective
3. CEA levels – too many false positives
4. Careful screening of high risk patients

SMALL BOWEL NEOPLASMS

Clinical features
1. Primary smalll bowel tumours are very rare
2. Approx. 75% are malignant
3. Vague symptoms lead to delayed diagnosis:
    a. Pain from intermittent obstruction
    b. Bleeding

Classification

Benign
1. Adenomata
2. Lipomata
3. Leiomyomata
4. Hamartomata: Peutz–Jegher syndrome
    (i) Autosomal dominant
    (ii) Intestinal polyposis, colonic polyps in 30%, hamartomata
    (iii) Malignant potential – there are rare examples of malignancy occurring in these polyps
    (iv) Melanin spots of the oral mucosa, palms and soles
    (v) Recurring bleeding or obstruction may necessitate local resection
5. Neurogenic, haemangiomata, lymphangiomata – all very rare

Malignant
1. Adenocarcinoma
2. Lymphoma
3. Sarcoma
4. Carcinoid tumours
   a. May occur where there are Kulschitzky cells
      (i) GI tract (stomach to anus)
         Appendix 45%
         Ileum 30%
         Rectum 17%
         Rarer sites, e.g. pancreas
      (ii) Outside GI tract, e.g. bronchus
   b. Potential to metastasize is related to size and site

	% metastasis
Appendix	3
Ileum	30
<1 cm	2
1–2 cm	50
>2 cm	80

   c. Appendiceal carcinoids are rarely multiple, however ileal carcinoids are multiple in 30%
   d. 30% of patients may have a co-existing second primary malignant neoplasm of a separate histological type
   e. Lesions tend to excite marked fibrous reaction. They are generally submucosal unless ulceration occurs
   f. Treatment
      (i) Incidental benign appendiceal carcinoid often removed during appendicectomy
      (ii) Formal cancer operation for malignant lesions, attempting to remove all gross disease. Patients may do very well for long periods

MALIGNANT CARCINOID SYNDROME

Biochemical basis is complex. Main abnormality is diversion of tryptophan to serotonin. Liver normally inactivates this to 5-HIAA, which is excreted in the urine, and forms basis of diagnostic test. Syndrome is seen with carcinoid metastatic to liver, or originating in sites not drained by portal vein, e.g. bronchus. In addition substances such as kallikrein, histamine, prostaglandins are produced, and play an unknown role

Clinical features

Transient
1. Flushing

2. Diarrhoea
3. Asthma

Permanent
1. Facial hyperaemia
2. Peripheral oedema
3. Pellagra (niacin is derived from tryptophan)
4. Valvular heart disease. Pulmonary and tricuspid

Treatment
1. Aggressive surgical resection where possible
2. Drugs
   (i) Antiserotonin agents – methysergide, cyproheptadine – good for bowel symptoms
   (ii) Somatostatin analogues will play increasing role.
   (iii) H_2 receptor blockers and steroids occasionally useful
   (iv) Chemotherapy: 5-FU and streptozotocin (tumour necrosis can cause a fatal crisis)

18. Inflammatory bowel disease

CROHN'S DISEASE

Pathological features
1. Transmural inflammatory disease
2. Thickened bowel, esp. submucosa with narrowed lumen, ulcerated nodular mucosa (cobblestone mucosa)
3. Mesenteric fat covering serosa
4. Enlarged mesenteric nodes
5. Non-caseating granulomata
6. Fistulization to neighbouring bowel
7. Skip lesions are common
8. May involve any part of the bowel from mouth to anus
   - (i) Small bowel only   30%
   - (ii) Ileocolitis   55%
   - (iii) Large intestine alone   15%

Clinical presentation
1. Abdominal pain
2. Partial small bowel obstruction
3. Diarrhoea
4. Fever
5. Fistulae – e.g. vaginal/vesical
6. Acute onset disease mimicking appendicitis with palpable mass in the right lower quadrant

Complications

Local
1. Obstruction
2. Perforation with abscess
3. Perianal abscess/fistula
4. Fistula – bowel, bladder, vagina

General
1. Malabsorption

2. Polyarthritis, ankylosing spondylitis
3. Erythema nodosum, pyoderma gangrenosum
4. Fatty liver, pericholangitis, portal fibrosis, gallstones
5. Uveitis
6. Periureteric fibrosis, right hydronephrosis
7. Carcinoma of the small and large bowel (20-fold increase)
8. Amyloidosis

Diagnosis
1. Barium studies showing narrowing (Kantor's string sign of terminal ileum), fistulae, skip lesions
2. Endoscopy
3. At laparotomy
4. CT scan

Medical management
1. Doctor–patient relationship is key
2. Symptomatic drugs for pain and diarrhoea – avoid addictive drugs
3. Iron and B_{12} replacement
4. Steroids, metronidazole, Salazopyrin (sulphasalazine) used in various combinations for active disease
5. No effective treatment available for maintaining remission
6. Immunosuppression for severe cases is being investigated (cyclosporin, Imuran)

Surgery

Concept of minimal surgery
1. There is no advantage of resecting anything more than grossly diseased small intestine. The recurrence rate is not decreased by resecting to microscopically clean margins
2. Stricturoplasty may avoid a resection in patients with multiple areas of narrowing

Types of operation
1. Small intestinal disease
   (i) Resection with primary reanastomosis
   (ii) Bypass of obstructed area, e.g. duodenum
   (iii) Stricturoplasty in patients at risk of developing short bowel syndrome
2. Illeocolitis
   Resection of diseased ileum and only that portion of the colon which is diseased, e.g. caecum, with reanastomosis
3. Large intestine disease
   (i) Ileorectal anastomosis. In young patients with rectal sparing – may delay need for permanent ileostomy

(ii) Panproctocolectomy with permanent ileostomy for extensive colonic and rectal involvement

Indications for surgery
1. Intractable symptoms despite optimal medical management
2. Obstruction which fails to resolve with suction
3. Abscess
4. Severe perianal disease
5. Complications of fistulae
6. Severe systemic complications

Results of surgery
1. Recurrence is a characteristic of Crohn's disease and colonoscopy within several weeks of resection and reanastomosis shows early signs of recurrent disease at the ileocolonic anastomosis in as many as 70%. Recurrence progresses at differing rates and some patients require reoperation
2. Frequency of symptomatic recurrence

30–40%	5 years
60%	10 years
75%	15 years

ULCERATIVE COLITIS

Pathological features
1. Primarily affects the mucosa and submucosa, with inflammatory cell infiltrate, crypt abscess, and ulcer formation
2. Redundant mucosa between ulcers forms pseudopolyps
3. Mucosa is friable and bleeds easily on contact
4. No skip areas
5. Rectosigmoid most commonly involved – 50% total colonic involvement
6. Chronic disease causes shortening and thickening of the bowel wall with haustral loss

Clinical presentation
1. May be fulminant, chronic, relapsing
2. Tenesmus, profuse diarrhoea, blood, pus, mucus
3. Dehydration and toxicity depending on form

Complications

Local
1. Perforation
2. Haemorrhage
3. Megacolon

    (i) Usually occurs with initial acute episode
   (ii) May be precipitated by barium enema, anticholinergics, morphine
  (iii) Suspect if patient with acute colitis has a sharp decrease in number of stools without improvement in general condition
  (iv) Abdominal distension may be only physical sign
   (v) X-ray shows dilated colon
  (vi) Risk of rupture increases in face of progressive dilatation

4. Stricture
5. Risk of carcinoma
    (i) Extent of disease: patients with extensive disease have greater risk than patients with left-sided disease
   (ii) Duration: after 10 years of disease, risk is about 2–3% per year. For first 7 years risk is minimal
  (iii) Onset: patients with onset of UC < 25 years have twice the incidence
  (iv) Carcinoma is frequently multiple, poorly differentiated, and presents with symptoms of colitis, therefore making early diagnosis difficult
   (v) 5-year survival rate is < 20%
  (vi) For patients who have had the disease for 10 years or longer regular colonoscopic surveillance is recommended. Any signs of dysplasia should lead to early colectomy

General
1. Weight loss, anaemia, hypoproteinaemia
2. Arthritis, ankylosing spondylitis
3. Iritis
4. Fatty liver hepatitis, cirrhosis
5. Pyoderma gangrenosum, erythema nodosum

Diagnosis
1. Exclude specific causes of diarrhoea, e.g. bacillary, amoebic
2. Sigmoidoscopy and biopsy
3. Differentiation from Crohn's disease – may be very difficult

Management of ulcerative colitis
1. Chronic ulcerative colitis
    (i) Control diarrhoea
   (ii) Salazopyrin
  (iii) Steroids. Mostly used for controlling acute episodes. Patients should be weaned off steroids as soon as an exacerbation of the disease is under control
  (iv) Newer agents, e.g. 5 ASA preparations
   (v) Attention to general nutrition, iron, and vitamins
2. Acute disease
    (i) May require hospital admission if poor response to outpatient therapy

    (ii) High dose corticosteroids
       a. Can mask perforation
       b. Increase the morbidity of surgery
    (iii) Nil by mouth. TPN may be required
    (iv) Cyclosporin – role under investigation

Surgery and ulcerative colitis

Elective surgery
1. Intractable symptoms
2. Long-standing active disease which increases risk of carcinoma

Emergency
Haemorrhage, perforation, toxic megacolon, or severe flares which
have failed course of high dose steroids, complete bowel rest, and
intravenous feeding

Types of operation
1. Subtotal colectomy with ileostomy
   a. Standard operation for acutely ill patient
   b. Most suitable initial operation if diagnosis of ulcerative colitis
      vs. Crohn's disease is uncertain
2. Panproctocolectomy and permanent ileostomy
   a. Low complication rate
   b. Permanent ileostomy unacceptable to some patients
3. Ileo-anal pouch operation
   a. Accompanied by greater complication rate
   b. Increasing incidence of pouchitis with time
   c. Avoids need for permanent ileostomy

COMPLICATION OF STOMAS (ILEOSTOMY OR COLOSTOMY)

1. Retraction
2. Stenosis
3. Prolapse
4. Parastomal hernia
5. Lateral space obstruction

19. Diverticular disease

PATHOPHYSIOLOGY

1. Postulated that a low residue diet leads to hypersegmentation and hypertrophy of circular muscle
2. Increased intraluminal pressure forms pulsion diverticula, which consist of an outpouching of mucosa alongside the antimesenteric tenia coli, close to a large penetrating vessel
3. Believed that dietary bran lowers intraluminal pressure, and may reduce the tendency for diverticulum formation
4. Incidence rises with age (65 years: 35%). Vast majority remain asymptomatic
5. Most common in the sigmoid and left colon, less commonly right

COMPLICATIONS

1. Bleeding. May be massive, without any signs of inflammation. Aortography has shown that most cases are due to haemorrhage from right-sided diverticula, even though they are more common on the left
2. Diverticulitis. May present as 'left-sided appendicitis'. Begins with perforation of a single diverticulum, and initial formation of a small pericolic abscess. This may resolve or progress to:
   (i) Formation of larger pericolic abscess
   (ii) Free perforation into peritoneum with resulting generalized peritonitis
   (iii) Perforation into adjacent bladder, bowel or vagina
3. Bowel obstruction
   (i) Large bowel – secondary to stricture
   (ii) Small bowel – secondary to adhesions

INVESTIGATIONS

1. Barium enema
   (i) Diverticulitis usually involves a long segment, vs. short in cancer
   (ii) Funnel-shaped transition from normal to diseased bowel

vs. abrupt transition in cancer
  (iii) Spasticity may be relieved by i.v. glucagon in diverticulitis
  (iv) Mucosa is normally intact in diverticulitis, and saw-tooth
       pattern may be seen
  (v) Intramural fistulae provide good evidence of diverticulitis
2. Colonoscopy
   Diverticular disease and colon carcinoma may co-exist
3. CT scan
   (i) In the acute setting CT may be very helpful to confirm
       diagnosis
   (ii) May enable percutaneous abscess drainage

MANAGEMENT

Acute diverticulitis
1. Many mild cases resolve spontaneously or with oral antibiotics
   and liquid diet
2. More severe cases require intravenous antibiotics
3. Surgery for cases with generalized peritonitis/failure to respond
   to antibiotics
   (i) Resection of diseased colon and creation of colostomy and
       mucous fistula/Hartman pouch
   (ii) Proximal colostomy if resection unsafe
   (iii) Drainage of abscess cavity if present

Haemorrhage
1. Most stop spontaneously
2. Red cell scan/arteriography for localization of bleeding site
3. Segmental resection if bleeding does not cease
4. Subtotal colectomy if bleeding cannot be localized

Chronic diverticulitis
1. Repeated attacks of pain typically in LLQ
   Elective resection
2. Stricture/obstruction
   Differentiation from carcinoma may be impossible until resection
   is complete
3. Fistula
   Colo-vesical is most common
   Excision of diseased bowel and fistula, with closure of healthy
   tissues

20. Perianal disease

CONDITIONS CAUSING ACUTE PERIANAL PAIN
1. Thrombosed haemorrhoids
2. Perianal haematoma
3. Fissure-in-ano
4. Perianal/rectal abscess
5. Proctalgia fugax

HAEMORRHOIDS

Complications
1. Bleeding
2. Mucous discharge and pruritus ani
3. Thrombosis
4. Ulceration

Treatment
1. Dietary bran
2. Suppositories for symptomatic relief
3. Rubber band ligation for internal haemorrhoids
4. Injection therapy
5. Controlled anal stretch
6. Haemorrhoidectomy – for combined internal–external haemorrhoids which cannot be banded

ANAL FISSURE

Clinical features
1. Presents with history of pain after bowel movements
2. Pain may last for hours
3. Bleeding – mostly on toilet paper

On examination
1. Sentinel skin tag
2. Hypertrophied anal papilla

3. Anal ulcer – typically occur in the posterior midline
4. Rectal examination may be impossible without causing severe pain, and may have to be performed under general anaesthesia
5. Atypical fissures may be seen in:
   (i) Crohn's disease
   (ii) Epidermal carcinoma
   (iii) Immunosuppressed patients
   (iv) Syphllis
   (v) TB

Treatment
1. Acute fissures
   (i) Warm soaks
   (ii) Stool softeners
2. Chronic fissures
   (i) Controlled anal stretch (4 fingers, 4 minutes)
   (ii) Lateral internal sphincterotomy

ANORECTAL ABSCESS AND FISTULA

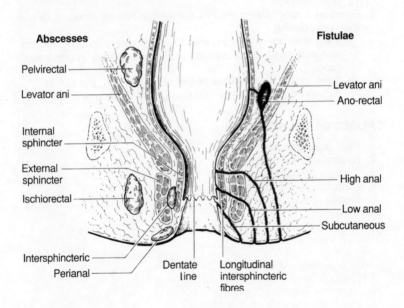

Abscesses

Pelvirectal

Levator ani

Internal sphincter

External sphincter

Ischiorectal

Intersphincteric

Perianal

Dentate line

Longitudinal intersphincteric fibres

Fistulae

Levator ani

Ano-rectal

High anal

Low anal

Subcutaneous

Pathology
1. Formation of abscess in anal gland between internal spincter and longitudinal intersphincteric muscle fibres
2. Pus tracks up/down to locations in diagram

3. Fistula is an inflammatory tract with external opening in the skin and internal opening in anal/rectal mucosa. Fistula originates in an abscess

Clinical features

Abscesses
1. Generally cause constant throbbing pain
2. Localized tenderness is present well before fluctuation
3. Drainage required – do not wait for fluctuation
4. At time of drainage attempt is made to locate internal opening and include it in the drainage to prevent recurrence

Fistulae
1. May follow drainage of an abscess if internal opening is not found
2. Present with chronic drainage and recurrent pain

Treatment
1. Should be laid open without damage to sphincter muscle – may be very complex
2. Goodsall's rule: relates the location of the internal opening to the external opening
   (i) If external opening is anterior to an imaginary line through the mid-anal canal, the fistula generally runs directly into the anal canal
   (ii) If the external opening is posterior to this line, the fistula curves into the posterior midline of the anal canal

CAUSES OF PRURITUS ANI
1. Poor anal hygiene
2. Redundant mucosa, fissures
3. Contact dermatitis, eczema
4. Diabetes, Hodgkin's disease
5. Monilia, pediculosis, worms
6. Idiopathic

21. Appendicitis

APPENDICITIS

Clinical features
1. Anorexia. Usually first sign – almost invariable
2. Pain. Initially central (visceral) then migrates (usually within 4–6 hours) to site of inflamed appendix (parietal)
   a. Retrocaecal: flank/back pain
   b. Pelvic: suprapubic pain, dysuria. (Tenderness on rectal examination)
   c. Postileal: testicular pain, diarrhoea
3. Vomiting
4. Fever. Initially low grade unless perforation
5. Foetor oris may be present
6. Rovsing's sign: pain in the RLQ with palpation in the LLQ – indicates parietal inflammation in RLQ
7. Psoas sign: right thigh extension causes pain from stretching the psoas muscle – indicates retrocaecal inflammation
8. Obturator sign: pain produced by passive internal rotation of the flexed right thigh – indicates inflammation near obturator internus muscle
9. Leukocytosis variable: should not influence diagnosis or management
10. In pregnancy the appendix may be displaced superiorly by the enlarging uterus, thus altering the point of maximal pain and tenderness
11. Atypical presentations may occur in very young and old

Complications
1. Rupture – more common after 24 hours, in very young and the elderly. Avoid delay in diagnosis
2. Abscess formation
3. Generalized peritonitis
   (i) Mucocoele
   (ii) Infertility – scarring of fallopian tubes
4. Pyelophlebitis and liver abscess – rare

Differental diagnosis
1. Acute mesenteric adenitis
2. Gastroenteritis
3. Regional enteritis or Yersiniosis
4. Urinary tract infection/renal colic
5. Pelvic inflammatory disease
6. Ovarian cyst complication (torsion, haemorrhage, rupture, incarceration)
7. Ruptured ectopic pregnancy
8. Perforated peptic ulcer
9. Perforated caecal carcinoma
10. Caecal diverticulitis
11. Cholecystitis
12. Diverticulitis
13. Testicular torsion
14. Meckel's diverticulitis
15. Henoch–Shönlein purpura
16. Basal pneumonia
17. Herpes zoster
18. Trauma: rectus sheath haematoma – history may be forgotten especially by children

In pregnancy appendix moves laterally and cephalad

Diagnostic tests
1. Diagnosis remains clinical. It is better to remove a normal appendix than allow perforation to occur
2. Elevated white cell count – unreliable
3. Barium enema for non-visualization of appendix – unreliable
4. Ultrasound – very operator dependent
5. Laparoscopy – used more frequently ± appendicectomy

Treatment
1. Preoperative resuscitation of sick patients to correct hypovolaemia, electrolyte disorders, diabetes
2. Acute appendicitis without rupture:
   Appendicectomy, perioperative antibiotics
3. Acute appendicitis ruptured with generalized peritonitis:
   Appendicectomy, peritoneal toilet, antibiotics (5–10 days)
4. Appendix abscess:
   Appendicectomy if feasible, drainage of abscess, antibiotics. Interval appendectomy depending on patient
5. Appendix mass evident on initial clinical examination in non-toxic patient:
   i.v. antibiotics, monitor size of mass. Most resolve. If systemic toxicity develops/mass enlarges – drain – interval appendectomy. Barium study/CT may be needed to exclude caecal carcinoma or Crohn's disease

6. It may sometimes be impossible to distinguish between an appendiceal phlegmon and a perforating caecal carcinoma. Under these conditions a right hemicolectomy may be required

CAUSES OF A MASS IN THE RIGHT LOWER QUADRANT

1. Appendicitis
2. Caecal carcinoma
3. Crohn's disease
4. Psoas abscess
5. Pelvic kidney
6. Ovarian cyst
7. Lymphoma
8. Aneurysm
9. Foreign body perforation
10. Caecal diverticulitis
11. TB, actinomycosis, amoebiasis

22. Peritonitis

PERITONITIS

Causes
1. Intra-abdominal viscus
   - (i) Appendicitis
   - (ii) Perforated peptic ulcer
   - (iii) Cholecystitis
   - (iv) Diverticulitis
   - (v) Ischaemic bowel
   - (vi) Anastomotic leak
   - (vii) Pancreatitis
   - (viii) Oesophageal rupture
   - (ix) Aortic rupture/dissection
   - (x) Iatrogenic: endoscopy, barium enema
2. Gynaecological
   - (i) Ovarian cyst complication
   - (ii) Ectopic pregnancy
   - (iii) Acute salpingitis
   - (vi) Postpartum infection
3. External source
   - (i) Penetrating trauma
   - (ii) Postoperative
   - (iii) Dialysis
   - (iv) Starch
4. Haematogenous spread
   - (i) Pneumococcal
   - (ii) Streptococcal
   - (iii) Staphylococcal
   - (iv) TB

Conditions which can mimic peritonitis
1. Diabetic ketoacidosis
2. Sickle cell crisis
3. Herpes zoster
4. Familial Mediterranean fever

5. Rectus sheath haematoma
6. Acute intermittent hepatic porphyria

Clinical features of peritonitis
1. Sharp pain: worse on movement of coughing
2. Pain may be referred to shoulder: diaphragmatic irritation
3. Vomiting and distension
4. Guarding and percussion/rebound tenderness
5. Diminished bowel sounds – unreliable
6. Pelvic peritonitis may present as diarrhoea, dysuria, frequency. Rectal examination – tenderness of the pelvic peritoneum
7. In elderly and patients on steroid therapy signs may be masked. A high index of suspicion is necessary

Diagnosis
1. Essentially a clinical diagnosis based on history and physical examination
2. Upright or lateral decubitus X-rays may reveal free air indicating perforation. Patient should be in position for 10 minutes prior to film
3. Peritoneal lavage may be useful in some cases

Course
1. Resolution – either spontaneous or with aid of antibiotics
2. Abscess formation
3. Generalized peritonitis
   (i) Systemic toxicity
   (ii) Sequestration of fluid within adynamic bowel and in peritoneal exudate
   (iii) Respiratory failure from diaphragm elevation and fixation, and septicaemia, leading to acidosis and hypoxaemia

Treatment
1. Diagnosis
2. Volume replacement, guided by CVP, haematocrit, urine output
3. Antibiotic therapy
4. Surgery for specific problems

INTRA-ABDOMINAL ABSCESS

Sites
1. Right and left subphrenic spaces
2. Subhepatic space
3. Lesser sac
4. Pouch of Douglas
5. Right and left paracolic gutters
6. Around diseased viscera, e.g.

(i) Periappendiceal
(ii) Pericholecystic
(iii) Pericolic
(iv) Tubo-ovarian
(v) Interloop

Clinical features
1. General malaise, fever, weight loss, failure to progress following surgery
2. May have hiccoughs or shoulder pain
3. May have a palpable mass per abdomen or rectum
4. Remember pus somewhere, pus nowhere, pus under the diaphragm
5. Patients may become jaundiced
6. Tend to be polymicrobial with anaerobes predominating
7. Elevated WBC, ESR, commonly seen

Investigations
1. Plain X-ray may show an air fluid level, or gas bubbles
2. Ultrasound – view often limited by bowel gas
3. CT scan – most useful

Treatment
1. Adequate drainage remains the cornerstone of treatment
2. Open or percutaneous methods depending on the location of the abscess, and the skill of the radiologist
3. Conditions for percutaneous drainage under CT or US guidance include:
   (i) Generally unilocular abscess
   (ii) Safe percutaneous route
   (iii) Joint evaluation by surgeon and radiologist
   (iv) Operative back-up must be available if percutaneous drainage fails
   (v) The catheter drain has to be regularly irrigated after placement to prevent blockage
   (vi) Appropriate antibiotics are used in conjunction with drainage

23. Intestinal obstruction

CAUSES

Mechanical

1. *Intraluminal*
    (i) Meconium
    (ii) Intussusception (see below)
    (iii) Gallstones
    (iv) Impaction, faecal, worms, barium, bezoar, food, e.g. citrus
        following gastroenterostomy

2. *Bowel wall*
    (i) Congenital
        a. Atresia, stenosis
        b. Imperforate anus
        c. Duplications
        d. Meckel's (see below)
    (ii) Traumatic
        a. Haematoma
        b. Stricture
    (iii) Inflammatory
        a. Crohn's disease
        b. Diverticulitis
    (iv) Neoplastic
    (v) Miscellaneous
        a. Potassium tablet-induced stricture
        b. Radiation
        c. Endometriosis

3. *Extraluminal*
    (i) Adhesions/bands
    (ii) Hernia
    (iii) Annular pancreas
    (iv) Anomalous vessels
    (v) Abscesses

(vi) Haematoma
(vii) Neoplasms
(viii)Volvulus (see below)

Non-mechanical (paralytic ileus)
1. Abdominal causes
    (i) Postoperative
    (ii) Peritonitis
    (iii) Vascular occlusion
2. Systemic causes
    (i) Electrolyte disorders: hypokalaemia, hypomagnesaemia
    (ii) Uraemia, diabetic coma
    (iii) Hypothyroidism
3. Drugs
    (i) Anticholinergic
    (ii) Opiates, e.g. morphine
4. Reflex
    (i) Plaster casts
    (ii) Postpartum
    (iii) Renal colic
    (iv) Retroperitoneal haemorrhage
    (v) Fractured vertebrae

CLASSIFICATION

General
1. Simple: without intestinal ischaemia
2. Strangulated: with intestinal ischaemia
3. Partial/complete

Location

Large bowel
1. Carcinoma ⎫
2. Diverticulitis ⎬   90%
3. Volvulus ⎭

Small bowel
1. Incarcerated hernia ⎫ 90% cases
2. Adhesions ⎭

MECHANICAL OBSTRUCTION

Symptoms
1. Pain: usually cramping. Constant pain suggests strangulation
2. Vomiting: early with high obstructions, late in low cases

3. Constipation – faeces and flatus

Signs
1. Dehydration depending on duration of obstruction
2. Abdominal distension, esp. with low obstructions
3. Tenderness: not necessarily present
4. Scars from prior operation: suggests adhesions
5. Incarcerated hernia: easy to miss in obese patients
6. Rectal examination: rectal cancer may be palpable, blood in stool

Investigation
1. Diagnosis is mainly on clinical grounds and may be missed by experienced surgeons if history is not typical
2. X-ray may show:
    (i)   Distended bowel: either large or small bowel with air-fluid levels
    (ii) No abnormality: closed loop obstruction (both limbs of loop are obstructed with risk of early ischaemia)
    (iii) Air in the biliary tree: gallstone ileus
    (iv) Contrast studies may confirm diagnosis in patients with unclear history. Not for routine use
3. CT scan. Although expensive may establish the diagnosis in certain patients in whom diagnosis is in doubt, and also identify unsuspected problems, e.g. abscess, metastases which may alter treatment. Not for routine use

Treatment
1. Volume and electrolyte replacement: the longer the period of obstruction the more fluid replacement is required to avoid intraoperative hypotension and its sequelae (MI, CVA, renal failure)
2. Decompression via nasogastric/long tube
    a. As part of initial resuscitation
    b. Treatment for partial obstruction which may resolve or allow time to prepare bowel for elective surgery
3. Surgery
    a. Complete small bowel obstruction: there is no reliable way to distinguish a simple from strangulating complete small bowel obstruction. Hence early operation is indicated to avoid bowel resection
    b. Complete small bowel obstruction in the presence of a competent ileocaecal valve and progressive caecal distension
    c. Partial small bowel obstruction: if patient fails to improve following a suitable period of nasogastric decompression. Period varies depending on condition of the patient, and cause of the partial obstruction

d. Partial large bowel obstruction: cause may be established by endoscopy in some patients, and patient can undergo bowel preparation to facilitate a single stage operation
e. Surgical procedures for intestinal obstruction
   (i) Lysis of adhesions
   (ii) Reduction/resection of intussusception
   (iii) Hernia reduction and repair
   (iv) Enterotomy − removal of gallstone or bezoar
   (v) Resection of obstructing lesion/strangulated bowel
   (vi) Bypass
   (vii) Untwisting of volvulus
   (viii) Decompression with proximal ostomy
      a. Ileostomy
      b. Caecostomy
      c. Colostomy

PARALYTIC IIEUS

Clinical features
1. Little or no abdominal pain
2. Abdominal distension
3. Failure to pass flatus/faeces
4. No local abdominal tenderness
5. Vomiting/persistently high nasogastric output
6. X-rays show gas throughout small and large bowel (does not exclude partial mechanical obstruction)

Treatment
1. Nasogastric suction
2. Treat cause
   (i) Correction of fluid/electrolyte/endocrine disorder
   (ii) Reduce analgesics
   (iii) Exclude causes which require surgery

INTUSSUSCEPTION

1. Children − 90% cases; no underlying cause
   (i) Children scream and become pale with colic
   (ii) Redcurrant jelly stool
   (iii) Sausage-shaped tumour palpable in most cases
   (iv) Barium reduction used to treat children
2. Adults: polyp, carcinoma, or Meckel's diverticulum is initiating factor
   (i) May present with intermittent bowel obstruction and palpable mass
   (ii) Resection generally required because of high incidence of organic cause

MECKEL'S DIVERTICULUM

1. Present in 2% population 2 ft (60 cm) above the ileocaecal valve. Most remain asymptomatic   *2 inches long*
2. May contain ectopic gastric or pancreatic tissue
3. Complications:
   - (i) 60% occur before 10 years
   - (ii) Diverticulitis
   - (iii) Bleeding ^{99m}Tc scan may be positive if the diverticulum contains heterotopic gastric mucosa
   - (iv) Obstruction
     - a. Intussusception
     - b. Volvulus
     - c. Vitello-intestinal band
   - (v) Perforation:
     a foreign body may get trapped

VOLVULUS

1. Sigmoid colon
   - (i) Typically elderly constipated patients
   - (ii) Rapid distension
   - (iii) X-ray shows 'bent inner tube'
   - (iv) Treatment
     - a. Rigid or flexible sigmoidoscopy can be diagnostic and therapeutic. Most cases can be reduced
     - b. High incidence of recurrence. Therefore elective sigmoid resection is advised
2. Caecum
   - (i) Associated with a persistent caecal mesentery
   - (ii) X-ray shows a large midabdominal loop
   - (iii) Early operation imperative because this is a closed loop and early strangulation likely
3. Small intestine
4. Rarely stomach and gallbladder

24. Liver

CAUSES OF HEPATOMEGALY IN SURGICAL PATIENTS

1. *Neoplastic*
   (i) Metastases
   (ii) Hepatoma
   (iii) Lymphoma

2. *Venous congestion*
   (i) Congestive cardiac failure
   (ii) Hepatic vein thrombosis

3. *Cirrhosis*

4. *Haemopoeitic*
   (i) Leukaemia
   (ii) Polycythaemia
   (iii) Myelofibrosis

5. *Inflammatory*
   (i) Hepatitis
   (ii) Hepatic abscess

6. *Congenital*
   (i) Reidel's lobe
   (ii) Polycystic disease

7. *Parasitic*
   (i) Amoebic hepatitis
   (ii) Hydatid

CLASSIFICATION OF JAUNDICE

1. *Prehepatic – haemolysis*
   (i) Blood transfusions
   (ii) Severe sepsis

(iii) Hereditary sperocytosis
(iv) G6PD deficiency

2. *Hepatic*
   (i) Hepatitis
  (ii) Cirrhosis
 (iii) Drugs
 (iv) Liver tumours

3. *Posthepatic (obstructive)*
   (i) Stone
  (ii) Stricture
 (iii) Tumour
     a. Pancreas
     b. Bile duct
     c. Nodes
 (iv) Pancreatitis

INVESTIGATION OF LIVER FUNCTION

1. *Liver function tests*
    (i) Serum bilirubin
   (ii) Alkaline phosphatase, GGT
  (iii) Coagulation tests (PT, PTT, fibrinogen)
  (iv) Transaminases
   (v) Blood sugar
  (vi) Blood ammonia
 (vii) Serum albumin

2. *Liver biopsy – complications*
   (i) Haemorrhage
  (ii) Bile leak
 (iii) Pneumothorax

3. *Ultrasound and CT*
   (i) Can detect metastases/abscess and guide biopsy
  (ii) Provide evidence for extrahepatic obstruction if there is ductal
     dilatation

4. *Scintillation scanning*
Used to detect intrahepatic lesions. Overalll not as helpful as
CT/US

5. *Percutaneous transhepatic cholangiography*
Provides details of biliary tract enabling differentiation between
hepatic and extrahepatic obstruction

6. *ERCP*
Enables biliary tract pathology to be identified and sometimes
treated, e.g. papillotomy for stone.

PYOGENIC LIVER ABSCESS

1. *Causes*
    (i) Ascending biliary infection
    (ii) Septicaemia
    (iii) Direct extension of intraperitoneal infection
    (iv) Trauma
    (v) Haematogenous infection via portal vein
    (vi) Idiopathic 20%

2. *Clinical presentation*
    (i) Fever is most common
    (ii) Jaundice is uncommon
    (iii) Liver enlargement, and tenderness may be present
    (iv) Alkaline phosphatase and WBC elevation common

3. *Treatment*
Percutaneous or open drainage plus antibiotics

AMOEBIC ABSCESS

1. *Pathology*
    (i) Amoebae gain access to portal vein via bowel ulcer
    (ii) Usually single lesions in the right lobe, containing 'anchovy
         paste'

2. *Clinical features*
    (i) Pain is seen early c.f. pyogenic abscess, and is related to the
         site of the abscess
    (ii) Causes tender liver
    (iii) Fever not as marked as pyogenic abscess

3. *Complications*
    (i) May rupture into:
         a. Pleura
         b. Lung
         c. Pericardium
         d. Peritoneum
         e. Colon
    (ii) May become secondarily infested (20%)

4. *Treatment*
    (i) Metronidazole
    (ii) Aspiration may be required

HYDATID DISEASE OF THE LIVER

(75% of hydatid cysts are in the liver)

1. Life cycle
   (i) Ova in sheep offal eaten by dogs
   (ii) Tapeworm develops in dog and sheds ova
   (iii) Ova on contaminated vegetable, etc. eaten by man
   (iv) Ingested ova penetrate stomach and reach liver

2. Hydatid cyst
   (i) 80% in right lobe
   (ii) Calcified rim on X-ray
   (iii) Casoni's test, and complement fixation test used

3. Complications
   (i) Rupture into pleura, biliary tree, peritoneal cavity, which may be accompanied by urticaria, and other anaphylactic manifestations
   (ii) Secondary infection

4. Treatment
   (i) Calcified cysts are inactive and require no treatment
   (ii) Others: aspiration, injection with hypertonic saline or peroxide, and excision
   (iii) There is no response to drug treatment

PHYSICAL STIGMATA OF LIVER DISEASE/FAILURE

1. Jaundice
2. Spider naevi
3. White nails
4. Dupuytren's contracture
5. Palmar erythema
6. Clubbing
7. Foetor hepaticus
8. Ascites
9. Slurred speech
10. Flapping tremor
11. Constructional apraxia
12. Hepatic coma
13. Parotid enlargement
14. Gynaecomastia
15. Testicular atrophy
16. Splenomegaly ⎫ with portal hypertension
17. Caput medusae ⎭

PORTAL HYPERTENSION

(Normal portal pressure is between 80–150 mm water)

Classification

1. *Hepatic*
   All forms of cirrhosis; accounts for 90% patients

2. *Prehepatic*
   Portal vein thrombosis
      (i) Umbilical sepsis/exchange transfusion
     (ii) Pyelophlebitis: appendicitis/diverticulitis
    (iii) Platelet disorder: myelofibrosis
    (iv) Pancreatic tumour

3. *Posthepatic*
      (i) Hepatic vein obstruction
     (ii) Constrictive pericarditis
    (iii) Budd–Chiari syndrome
    (iv) Veno-occlusive disease

Complications
1. Hypertrophy of portosystemic collaterals
      (i) Oesophageal varices
     (ii) Haemorrhoids
    (iii) Caput medusae
    (iv) Other intra-abdominal varices which make surgery difficult
2. Splenomegaly: can lead to hypersplenism
3. Ascites
4. Hepatic failure

Clinical course of oesophageal varices
1. 30% patients with varices bleed
2. Following a bleed there is a 60% chance of a recurrence
3. Cirrhotics who bleed have a 70% mortality within a year
4. Prophylactic shunting in patients who have not bled is not
   advised because there is no way of predicting who will bleed,
   and encephalopathy may be induced.
5. In adult patients with varices, upper intestinal bleeding is due to:
     a. Varices   50%
     b. Gastritis   30%
     c. Peptic ulcer 10%

Management of oesophageal varices

1. *Non-operative*
     (i) Volume replacement

a. Fresh blood (less ammonia)
b. Clotting factors
c. Enemas   } to reduce nitrogen
d. Neomycin and lactulose } load to liver
 (ii) Balloon therapy. Sengstaken–Blakemore tube
a. Asphyxiation ⎫
b. Aspiration   ⎬ complications
c. Ulceration   ⎭
(iii) Endoscopic sclerosis of varices
a. Controls bleeding in up to 90% cases, and can be
   repeated
b. Has greatly reduced the need for emergency shunts
(iv) Drug therapy
a. Vasopressin. Systemic works as well as local infusion –
   contraindicated in coronary disease
b. Propranolol. Lowers portal pressure and seems to have a
   long-term beneficial effect

2. *Operative*
(i) Survival is increased if (Child's criteria):
a. Albumin is > 25 g/l (2.5 g/100 ml)
b. Bilirubin < 34 µmol/l (2 mg/100 ml)
c. No ascites
d. Normal prothrombin time
e. No signs of encephalopathy
(ii) Emergency surgery to stop bleeding (50% mortality rate)
a. Portacaval shunt, provides best control
b. Transoesophageal ligation of varices/oesophagogastric
   devascularization have been tried in patients thought to be
   too ill for a shunt
(iii) Elective surgery
a. Carries lower mortality
b. Selective shunt – spares blood flow to the liver, in the
   hopes of reducing the incidence of encephalopathy, e.g.
   Warren distal speno-renal shunt
c. Underlying problem however is a poorly functioning liver,
   often in alcoholics with complex social situations
d. Surgery alters the mode of death from bleeding to
   encephalopathy but does not increase life span
e. Liver transplant may emerge as the best treatment

NEOPLASTIC DISEASE OF THE LIVER

Classification
1. Primary
   (i) Hepatoma
   (ii) Cholangiocarcinoma

        (iii) Adenoma – oral contraceptive
  2. Secondary (most common)
        (i) From portal spread
        (ii) Systemic: lung, breast, etc.
        (iii) Direct: stomach, colon, gallbladder

Hepatoma   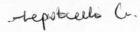 _Hepatcells C._

Aetiology
  1. Cirrhosis
  2. Hepatitis B & C
  3. Haemochromatosis
  4. Aflatoxin – dietary

Clinical features
  1. Weight loss, malaise
  2. Pain following necrosis or haemorrhage
  3. Hepatomegaly
  4. Ascites
  5. Jaundice is common
  6. 30% have signs of portal hypertension
  7. Rapid increase in signs/symptoms of cirrhosis/
     haemochromatosis
  8. Hypoglycaemia or improvement of diabetes
  9. Alpha-fetoprotein   _α FP._
        (i) 70% positive in Africa
        (ii) 30% positive in West
        (iii) May be positive in any regenerative liver condition
 10. Resection is only hope of cure at present, but only performed
     for localized non-metastatic cases

Clinical features of metastases in liver
  1. Large hard irregular liver
  2. Jaundice
  3. Liver failure
  4. Ascites
  5. IVC obstruction with leg oedema
  6. Resection of 'solitary' liver metastases is being performed
     increasingly frequently

LIVER TRAUMA
  1. Increased incidence with high speed injuries
  2. 75% have additional abdominal injuries, e.g. spleen
  3. Nearly 50% have thoracic injuries
  4. Present with:
        (i) Shock 75% cases

(ii) Upper abdominal pain very common
5. Diagnosis
    (i) Clinical suspicion
    (ii) Peritoneal lavage
    (iii) Abdominal CT scan
6. Treatment
    (i) Treat shock and associated thoracic injuries
    (ii) Direct control of bleeding vessels if possible
    (iii) Remove all necrotic tissue
    (iv) Lobectomy for massive damage
    (v) Hepatic artery ligation may have a place in selected cases, but most bleeding occurs from hepatic veins
    (vi) Occasionally bleeding cannot be controlled and the upper abdomen is packed for 24 hours. A second operation is then performed to remove the packing. This may be life-saving
    (vii) Provide adequate drainage
    (viii) Avoid suturing of lacerations. This produces fluid filled dead space. Contents may ultimately rupture into biliary tree causing haemobilia or become infected

25. Gallbladder and bile ducts

GALLSTONES

Classification

1. *Cholesterol stones*
   - (i) 75% cholestrol by weight
   - (ii) Usually contain a pigmented centre
   - (iii) About 75% of human gallstones

2. *Pigment stones forming in gallbladder*
   - (i) Usually black and hard
   - (ii) Composed of calcium bilirubinate and pigment polymers
   - (iii) 50% are visible on abdominal films
   - (iv) Bile is usually sterile

3. *Pigment stones formed in bile ducts*
   - (i) Dull reddish-brown to black
   - (ii) Composed of calcium bilirubinate and calcium soaps of fatty acids
   - (iii) Usually form in infected bile
   - (iv) Soft and friable

Predisposing factors

1 *Cholesterol stones*
   - (i) Obesity
   - (ii) Oestrogen effect on cholesterol secretion:
     - a. Contraceptive pill
     - b. Pregnancy
   - (iii) Diabetes
   - (iv) Inflammatory bowel disease (reduced availability of bile salts)

2. *Pigment stones*
   - (i) Most are idiopathic
   - (ii) Cirrhosis

(iii) Haemolysis
(iv) Total parenteral nutrition
(v) Bacteria in bile
(vi) Parasites – *Clonorchis, Ascaris*

Complications
1. Biliary colic
2. Acute cholecystitis
   Differential diagnosis
      (i) Peptic ulcer
      (ii) Pancreatitis
      (iii) Appendicitis
      (iv) Hepatitis
      (v) Myocardial infarction
      (vi) Pneumonia
      (vii) Pleurisy
      (viii) Herpes zoster
3. Chronic cholecystitis
4. Gallstone pancreatitis
5. Obstructive jaundice secondary to common duct stone.
   Courvoisier's rule: if in the presence of painless jaundice, the
   gallbladder is palpable, then a stone is not a likely cause
6. Cholangitis
   Clinical features
      (i) Jaundice
      (ii) Intermittent fever } Charcot's triad
      (iii) Rigors
7. Fistulization from the biliary tree to stomach, duodenum, small
   bowel or colon
8. Perforation of the gallbladder and peritonitis
9. Carcinoma of the gallbladder, esp. with porcelain gallbladder

Investigations

1. *Plain abdominal X-ray*
   a. 10% of all calculi are radio-opaque
   b. Gas in biliary tree indicates biliary enteric fistula or infection
      with gas-forming organisms

2. *Ultrasound*
   a. Over 90% accurate
   b. Has become primary test for gallstones

3. *Isotope scanning*
   a. HIDA/PIPIDA gamma emitters
   b. Visualization of gallbladder rules out cholecystitis
   c. False positives may occur, e.g. patients who have not eaten
      for a few days
   d. May be used in jaundiced patients

4. *Endoscopic retrograde cholangiopancreatography (ERCP)*
   a. Provides details of pancreatico-biliary tree
   b. May be used to place a common bile duct stent
   c. May be used to retrieve common bile duct stones
   d. Tumour biopsy
   e. Complications:
      (i) Pancreatitis
      (ii) Perforation of common duct

5. *CT scan*
   Defines extent of tumour or pancreatitis

6. *Percutaneous transhepatic cholangiography*
   a. Delineates anatomy prior to exploring a patient with extrahepatic biliary obstruction who is unsuitable for ERCP
   b. Decompression of the biliary tree with a stent

7. *Choledochoscopy*
   Used intraoperatively to retrieve stones from the common bile duct

8. *Intra-operative ultrasound*
   Not used widely, but will probably have a greater role in the future

9. *Oral (OCG) and intravenous cholangiography (IVC)*
   a. OCG may occasionally be used if an US is normal and the patient has a very good history for gallstones. In combination with CCK it may help define rare motility disorders of the biliary tree. Also used to assess suitability for dissolution of gallstones
   b. IVC may be used to screen patients for common duct stones prior to laparoscopic cholecystectomy

CHOLECYSTITIS

Management
1. Early operation has been shown to decrease the overall time in hospital, and is accompanied by the same low mortality and morbidity rate as elective operation
2. Delayed cholecystectomy may be indicated if a patient presents late in the course of the illness and settles down on antibiotics
3. Emergency cholecystectomy is indicated
   (i) If patient shows signs of generalized peritonitis
   (ii) In cases of emphysematous cholecystitis

Type of operation

Laparoscopic cholecystectomy
1. Has rapidly evolved as the procedure of choice

2. Is not suitable for all cases
    (i) Prior surgery resulting in extensive adhesions
    (ii) Advanced cholecystitis
    (iii) Safety in pregnant patient still in some doubt
3. Surgeon must be prepared to convert to open operation if the anatomy is unclear, in order to minimize complications
4. Ongoing debate on the need for routine intra-operative cholangiography for the detection of common duct stones
5. Future instrument improvements will facilitate laparoscopic common duct exploration which is not widely available. Presently patients with suspected common bile duct stones undergo ERCP or open operation

Open operation
1. Very safe
2. Accompanied by incisional pain which delays recovery

Cholecystostomy
Open operation/percutaneous
1. If the gallbladder is too diseased to remove safely
2. If the patient is considered too ill to undergo major surgery

INDICATIONS TO EXPLORE THE COMMON BILE DUCT

1. Jaundice
2. Palpable stones in the common duct
3. Dilated common duct (> 12 mm) unless the operative cholangiogram is very good quality
4. Operative cholangiogram suggesting stones

COMPLICATIONS OF BILIARY SURGERY

Frequently arise from failure to recognize vascular or ductal anomalies which are extremely common in this area. To prevent inadvertent injury to the common duct, nothing is tied off at operation until the cystic—common duct junction is clearly seen. Specifically:
1. Jaundice: missed stone, ligature of common duct
2. Pancreatitis
3. Stricture of common bile duct
4. Recurrent cholangitis

MANAGEMENT OF RETAINED COMMON DUCT STONES

1. Extraction via T-tube
2. Endoscopic papillotomy

ASYMPTOMATIC GALLSTONES

1. Most should probably not be treated
2. Identification of patients who may be at greater risk of complications if they develop cholecystitis include:
   (i) Diabetics
   (ii) Patients on steroids, e.g. for inflammatory bowel disease
   (iii) Immunosuppressed patients
   (iv) Patients undergoing prolonged parenteral nutrition
   (v) Patients who live in remote regions or who travel frequently
3. Provided everything else is stable it is reasonable to remove the gallbladder if a patient is undergoing laparotomy for another reason

26. Pancreas

ANATOMY

1. Main duct of Wirsung joins the common bile duct at the papilla of Vater
2. Minor duct of Santorini joins the main duct in the neck of the pancreas and drains into the duodenum via the minor papilla
3. In 5–10% of patients duct of Santorini provides main drainage – pancreas divisum

ACUTE PANCREATITIS

Causes
1. Gallstones
2. Alcoholism
3. Trauma
4. Postoperative
     (i) Biliary surgery
     (ii) ERCP
     (iii) Gastrectomy
     (iv) Splenectomy
     (v) Afferent loop obstruction
5. Hyperlipidaemia
6. Thiazides, frusemide, steroids
7. Hypothermia
8. Viral: mumps, coxsackie
9. Hyperparathyroidism – probably not a cause but frequently listed as such
10. Miscellaneous: polyarteritis nodosa, malignant hypertension

Clinical features
1. Epigastric pain radiating to the back, often partially relieved by leaning forwards, and worse on lying back
2. Vomiting
3. Epigastric tenderness
4. Jaundice, glycosuria

5. Signs of hypovolemia (low BP, tachycardia)
6. Hypocalcaemia – rarely with carpopedal spasm
7. Flank (Grey Turner's) and periumbilical (Cullen's) ecchymosis seen in haemorrhagic pancreatitis

Diagnosis
Essentially a clinical diagnosis based on history and physical examination. To be differentiated from conditions with similar clinical and laboratory results, but which require urgent surgery
1. Amylase measurements
   a. Peak amylase occurs about one hour after the attack, and patients are frequently first seen after this
   b. Other diseases can lead to amylase elevation
        (i) Penetrating duodenal ulcer
        (ii) Perforated duodenal ulcer
        (iii) Acute cholecystitis
        (iv) Ischaemic bowel
        (v) Myocardial infarction
        (vi) Dissecting aortic aneurysm
        (vii) Ectopic pregnancy
        (viii) Afferent loop obstruction
2. Ultrasound may reveal gallstones
3. CT scan
        (i) Peripancreatic oedema
        (ii) Pancreatic necrosis
        (iii) Early pseudocyst formation

Management
1. Fluid replacement to avoid renal failure
2. Blood, insulin, and calcium supplements may be required
3. Repeated physical examination to ensure response to treatment and avoid delay in diagnosis of surgically correctable conditions
4. Control of pain
5. Nasogastric tube is useful if the patient is vomiting, but it probably does not alter course of illness
6. Antibiotics: no evidence that prophylactic antibiotics prevent the development of pancreatic abscess
7. Drugs: Trasylol, anticholinergics – no proven benefit
8. Laparotomy reserved for those cases which do not improve or if the diagnosis is in doubt
9. Surgical management of associated biliary tract disease
        (i) Optimal timing of surgery is controversial. Most wait if patient is improving, and carry out elective operation within a few weeks
        (ii) ERCP with clearance of common bile duct followed by laparoscopic cholecystectomy
        (iii) Open cholecystectomy, cholangiography ± common bile duct exploration

Complications
1. Pseudocysts
     (i) Rarely appear before the end of the second week
    (ii) More common after alcoholic pancreatitis
   (iii) May present with pain, fever, and persistent amylase elevation
   (iv) Most are diagnosed by CT scan when a patient does not completely improve following acute pancreatitis
    (v) Small cysts may resolve
   (vi) Untreated cysts may bleed or get infected
  (vii) Large persistent cysts are allowed to 'mature' for 6 weeks, and then drained
         a. By percutaneous aspiration
         b. By endoscopic internal drainage, e.g. cyst jejunostomy
         c. By internal drainage at open operation
2. Abscess
   a. Usually at least 3 weeks after the onset of pancreatitis
   b. Diagnosis
       (i) Swinging fever
      (ii) Positive blood cultures
     (iii) Gas bubbles on CT scan
     (iv) CT-guided aspiration of suspicious areas of necrosis may provide a means of making an earlier diagnosis
   c. Treatment
       (i) Involves extensive removal of all necrotic infected material
      (ii) May require several operations
With this aggressive approach mortality rate has been much decreased
3. Renal and respiratory failure
4. Thrombosis or rupture of portal or mesenteric vessels
5. Perforation of stomach or duodenum

CHRONIC PANCREATITIS

Clinical features
1. May be asymptomatic (calcification on X-ray)
2. Recurrent/continuous pain
3. Frequent association with alcohol and narcotic abuse
4. May cause obstructive jaundice
5. Steatorrhoea
6. Diabetes

Diagnosis
1. ERCP – ductal abnormalities
2. CT scan

Management
1. Correction of biliary disease if present

2. Abstinence from alcohol
3. Pancreaticojejunostomy if duct is dilated, subtotal pancreatectomy if duct is small

PANCREATIC TRAUMA

Clinical features
1. May be blunt or penetrating
2. Frequently overlooked because physical findings may be minimal
3. 80% have elevated amylase
4. CT ± ERCP may be useful in diagnosis

Treatment
1. Requires laparotomy to exclude major duct injury and provide drainage
2. Partial pancreatectomy may be required in severe cases

Complications
1. Fistula
2. Pseudocyst
3. Infection
4. Delayed haemorrhage

ZOLLINGER–ELLISON SYNDROME

Pathophysiology
1. Non β-islet cell tumour secreting gastrin
2. 60% are malignant
3. 20% associated with pituitary, parathyroid lesions (MEA 1)

Clinical features
1. Fulminant peptic ulcer often in atypical area, e.g. 3rd/4th part of duodenum or jejunum
2. Fulminant diarrhoea may also occur
3. Rugal hypertrophy

Diagnosis
1. Elevated gastrin
2. High basal acid secretory rate
3. Positive secretin test
4. CT may show pancreatic mass

Treatment
1. Gastrectomy
   a. Total gastrectomy
   b. Parietal cell vagotomy with H_2 blockers or omeprozole

2. Remove as much metastatic tumour as possible

INSULINOMA

Pathophysiology
1. β-islet cell tumour
2. Malignant 10%
3. Multiple 10%

Clinical features: Whipple's triad
1. Attacks precipitated by fasting or exercise
2. Fasting blood sugar of < 50 mg/ml
3. Relief of symptoms with glucose

Diagnosis
1. Insulin elevation in presence of hypoglycaemia
2. Preoperative localization studies using CT, angio, and selective venous sampling are variably successful

Treatment
1. Diazoxide for preoperative control of blood sugar
2. Surgery
   a. Complete pancreatic exploration
   b. Removal of tumour
   c. Intraoperative ultrasound may help localize tumour
3. Streptozotocin for functioning metastases

PANCREATIC CARCINOMA

Clinical features
1. Majority are ductal adenocarcinoma – poor prognosis is related to late presentation of adenocarcinoma. 80% have lymph node involvement or liver metastases
2. Cystadenocarcinomas are much less common but have a better prognosis
3. Head of pancreas is most commonly involved (60%)
4. Malaise and weight loss extremely common
5. Progressive jaundice especially with head lesions
6. Pain is present in over 50% cases, i.e. painless jaundice is rather unusual
7. 30% have palpable gallbladder

Diagnosis
1. CT scan plus or minus fine needle aspiration
2. ERCP
3. Tumour marker CA 19–9

Treatment
1. Resectable lesions:
   a. Pancreaticoduodenectomy (Whipple). Provides the only means of cure, but the number of patients who are cured is small. Using modern techniques this operation can be performed with a low (< 5% or better) mortality
   b. Roles of intraoperative radiation therapy and adjuvant chemotherapy being investigated
2. Unresectable lesion
   a. Asymptomatic jaundiced patient. Consider doing nothing.
   b. Symptomatic patient
      (i) Pruritus
          Biliary drainage – preferably endoscopic
      (ii) Gastric outlet obstruction:
           Gastrojejunostomy (does not always work) ± biliary drainage if required
      (iii) Pain:
            Percutaneous coeliac axis block

27. Spleen

CAUSES OF SPLENOMEGALY

1. Infections
   (i) Bacterial: typhoid
   (ii) Viral: mononucleosis
   (iii) Parasitic: hydatid
   (iv) Protozoal: malaria, schistosomiasis
2. Lymphoreticular
   (i) Hodgkin's
   (ii) Leukaemia (chronic myeloid, esp.)
   (iii) Polycythaemia
   (iv) Myeloid metaplasia
3. Portal hypertension
4. Cysts, abscess, tumour of spleen
5. Metabolic etc., e.g. amyloid, Gaucher's

SPLENIC RUPTURE

Types
1. Penetrating trauma
   (i) Transabdominal
   (ii) Transthoracic
2. Non-penetrating trauma
   (i) Immediate rupture 90%
   (ii) Delayed. Most are in fact delayed diagnosis
   (iii) Splenic rupture is most common injury following non-penetrating abdominal trauma
   (iv) 30% isolated injury
3. Operative trauma. Most can be repaired
4. Spontaneous rupture – minor trauma to pathologically enlarged or delicate spleen, e.g. mononucleosis, pregnancy

Clinical features
1 History of trauma
   a. May be forgotten by patient, especially children

   b. May be trival
2. Signs of hypovolaemia or tachycardia
3. Epigastric pain and tenderness 30%
4. Pain referred to the shoulder (esp. Trendelenburg position)
5. Signs may be minimal/absent initially

Diagnosis
1. Repeated physical examination
2. Serial haematocrit measurements
3. Peritoneal lavage in selected cases
4. Abdominal CT scan
5. Liver spleen scan
6. Plain abdominal X-ray findings are all unreliable and insensitive,
   but may be looked for
   (i) Fracture left lower ribs (this is a clinical diagnosis)
   (ii) Increased size of splenic shadow
   (iii) Medial displacement of gastric air bubble
   (iv) Depression of splenic flexure
   (v) Elevation and immobility of left diaphragm
7. Leukocytosis and thrombocytosis are unreliable

SPLENECTOMY

Indications
1. Trauma – if attempts to repair spleen fail
2. Blood disorders
   (i) Idiopathic thrombocytopoenic purpura (ITP)
   (ii) Hereditary spherocytosis
3. Staging of Hodgkin's disease
4. Primary splenic tumour, cyst, abscess
5. Part of another operation, e.g. radical gastrectomy

Complications
1. Haemorrhage
2. Acute dilatation of the stomach
3. Left lower lobe collapse
4. Pancreatitis/pseudocyst/abscess
5. Subphrenic abscess
6. Splenic vein thrombosis
7. Postoperative deep venous thrombosis and pulmonary embolism
8. Overwhelming post-splenectomy infection
   a. Mostly in children and immunosuppressed patients
   b. Patients undergoing elective splenectomy are given vaccine
      to reduce pneumococcal and *H. influenzae* infections
   c. Repair of ruptured spleen rather than removal if possible

28. Hernias

AETIOLOGY

1. Congenital/primary
2. Secondary to raised intra-abdominal pressure
   (i) Cough
   (ii) Constipation
   (iii) Cysts
   (iv) Carcinoma
   (v) Pregnancy
   (vi) Bladder outlet syndrome
3. Iatrogenic – incisional especially following midline incisions

PATHOLOGICAL ANATOMY

1. Sac – peritoneal diverticulum
2. Contents include:
   (i) Omentum
   (ii) Bowel: whole or part of circumference
   (iii) Bladder/bladder diverticulum
   (iv) Ovary ± fallopian tube
   (v) Appendix
   (vi) Meckel's diverticulum
   (vii) Fluid (ascites)
3. Coverings – the layers of the abdominal wall through which the sac passes

GENERAL CLASSIFICATION

1. *Reducible*
   (i) Contents of sac can be completely returned to abdominal cavity
   (ii) Cough impulse present
   (iii) May only be evident on examination of the patient standing

2. *Irreducible/incarcerated*
   (i) Contents of sac cannot be completely returned to the

peritoneal cavity
(ii) Cough impulse may or may not be present
(iii) Painless and non-tender

3. *Strangulated*
   a. Symptoms
      (i) Sudden onset of pain in a hernia
      (ii) Central colicky abdominal pain
      (iii) Vomiting
      (iv) Constipation
      (v) Abdominal distension
   b. Signs
      (i) Skin overlying hernia may become red
      (ii) Tense tender irreducible hernia
      (iii) No cough impulse
      (iv) Bowel sounds increased
   c. Differentiate from:
      (i) Torsion of testis
      (ii) Tender lymphadenitis
   d. Most common with:
      (i) Femoral hernia
      (ii) Indirect inguinal hernia
      (iii) Umbilical hernia

4. *Sliding*
   A portion of the hernia sac is composed of an organ such as the
   caecum on the right or the sigmoid colon on the left

INGUINAL CANAL

A musculo-aponeurotic defect, 1½" (4 cm) long, above and parallel
to the inguinal ligament, extending from the deep to the superficial
inguinal rings. Transmits the vas deferens in the male and the round
ligament in the female

1. *Deep ring*
   Lies a finger's breadth above the mid-inguinal point in the fascia
   transversalis lateral to the inferior epigastric vessels

2. *Superficial ring*
   Lies supero-medial to the pubic tubercle in external oblique
   aponeurosis

3. *Anterior wall*
   (i) Skin and superficial fascia
   (ii) External oblique aponeurosis
   (iii) Internal oblique aponeurosis

4. *Posterior wall*
    (i) Fascia transversalis
    (ii) Conjoint tendon medially

5. *Above*
   Fibres of the internal oblique and transversus arching over to form the conjoint tendon

6. Below
   Inguinal ligament

FEMORAL CANAL

The most medial compartment of the femoral sheath extending from the femoral ring to the saphenous opening
  1. Anterior: inguinal ligament
  2. Posterior: ligament of Astley Cooper
  3. Medial: lacunar ligament ± accessory obturator artery
  4. Lateral: femoral vein
  5. Contents: Cloquet's lymph node

CLASSIFICATION OF GROIN HERNIAS

1. *Indirect inguinal*
    (i) Sac is within the coverings of the spermatic cord, and as the hernia enlarges it traverses the inguinal canal from deep to superficial ring, and may eventually reach the scrotum
    (ii) Congenital in origin, i.e. patency of processus vaginalis
    (iii) Common cause of strangulated hernia
    (iv) The most common groin hernia

2. *Direct inguinal*
    (i) Hernia sac protrudes through a weakness in the fascia transversalis medial to the inferior epigastric vessels (Hesselbach's triangle). Borders of Hesselbach's triangle
       a. Lateral   inferior epigastric artery
       b. Medial   rectus sheath
       c. Inferior   inguinal ligament
    (ii) Very rarely strangulate because the neck of the sac is wide
    (iii) Bladder may be contained medially
    (iv) Rare in women
    (v) It is difficult to differentiate a direct from an indirect hernia clinically

3. *Femoral hernia*
    (i) Protrude through the femoral canal
    (ii) Most likely groin hernia to become strangulated

(iii) Usually small and therefore easily missed in the obese
(iv) The sac may contain part of the circumference of a piece of
bowel resulting in an ischaemic knuckle (Richter's hernia)
    a. Symptoms of gastroenteritis: diarrhoea and abdominal
       pain
    b. Strangulates early
    c. Late diagnosis because the patient may not have an easily
       palpable hernia
(v) More common in women

Distinguishing between groin hernias
1. Inguinal hernia lies above the inguinal ligament
2. Femoral hernia lies below and lateral to the inguinal ligament
3. The tip of a large femoral hernia may lie above the ligament due
to upward displacement by the attachment of the superficial
fascia to the saphenous opening. However:
  (i) The neck of the sac lies below the inguinal ligament
  (ii) Invagination of the scrotal skin with the examining finger
     reveals an empty inguinal canal

OTHER TYPES OF HERNIA

Umbilical hernia

1. Exomphalos
  (i) Present at birth
  (ii) Requires surgical repair

2. Congenital umbilical hernia
  (i) Mostly close spontaneously during the first year of life
  (ii) Surgical repair at 2 years if persistent

3. Umbilical hernia in adults
  (i) Especially in obese multiparous women
  (ii) Narrow neck, therefore liable to strangulate
  (iii) Often irreducible because of adhesions within the sac
  (iv) Contents of sac often include:
    a. Pre-peritoneal fat
    b. Omentum
    c. Transverse colon
    d. Small bowel

Epigastric hernia
1. Fatty protrusions through linea alba defect
2. Pain may be confused with dyspepsia

Obturator hernia
1. Herniation through the obturator canal
2. Especially in thin, elderly females
3. Narrow neck, therefore liable to strangulate
4. Richter type hernia may occur
5. Pain referred along the medial aspect of the thigh
6. May be felt per rectum/vagina
7. Easily forgotten cause of intestinal obstruction
8. May present as an abscess on the medial aspect of the thigh which drains faeculent material on incision

Spigelian hernia
1. Herniation via the arcuate line into the rectus sheath
2. Soft tender mass to one side of the lower abdominal wall

Incisional hernia
1. Predisposing factors
    (i) Midline vertical incisions
    (ii) Sutures tied too tight or too near the edge
    (iii) Obesity
    (iv) Cachexia and advanced malignant disease
    (v) Steriods
    (vi) Marked postoperative distension
2. Most begin early in the postoperative period
3. A serosanguinous wound discharge around the 10th postoperative day may signify a dehiscence and is an indication for careful palpation of the wound to determine if the fascial edges are still apposed

Rare hernias
1. Lumbar
2. Gluteal
3. Sciatic
4. These should be differentiated from:
    (i) Lipoma
    (ii) Fibrosarcoma
    (iii) Rare tuberculous abscess

GENERAL PRINCIPLES IN TREATMENT OF HERNIAS

1. Preoperative attention to smoking, weight reduction
2. Investigation and treatment of urinary outlet obstruction or colonic obstruction before hernia repair
3. A gentle attempt to reduce an incarcerated hernia may be worthwhile. There is a small risk of reduction 'en masse' i.e., lump disappears but contents remain incarcerated in sac. Unrecognized strangulated bowel may also be reduced

4. Attempted reduction of a strangulated hernia is completely contraindicated
5. Patients presenting with bowel obstruction, must be adequately resuscitated prior to repair
6. Principles of hernia repair
   (i) Identification of sac and contents, mobilization of sac, reduction of contents, ligation of sac
   (ii) Repair of fascial defect. Healthy tissue must be approximated without tension. There are numerous types of repair and personal preference dictates which is performed
       a. Shouldice
       b. Bassini
       c. Cooper's ligament
       d. Tension free method using mesh
       e. Laparoscopic hernia repair
7. Trusses are of little or no value

DIFFERENTIAL DIAGNOSIS OF A LUMP IN THE GROIN

1. Hernia
2. Lymph node
3. Saphena varix
4. Lipoma
5. Femoral aneurysm
6. Psoas abscess
7. Ectopic testicle
8. Hydrocoele of the canal of Nuck

29. Adrenal glands

ANATOMY

1. Arterial supply:
   (i) Inferior phrenic
   (ii) Aorta
   (iii) Renal artery
2. Venous drainage:
   (i) Left adrenal to renal vein
   (ii) Right adrenal to inferior vena cava
3. Weight 3.5–5.0 g

PHYSIOLOGY

Adrenal cortex
Coelomic mesothelial origina. Secretes:
1. Aldosterone (zona glomerulosa)
   Release stimulated by:
   Decrease in blood volume
   Increase in serum K^+
   Angiotensin-2
   ACTH
   Actions:
   Stimulates renal tubular absorption of K^+, Na^+
   H^+, NH_4^+
   Antagonist: Spironolactone
2. Cortisol (zona fascicularis)
   Diurnal rhythm (max a.m. min p.m.)
   Release stimulated by:
   Generally stressful stimuli, e.g. pain, hypoglycaemia
   Actions:
   Hyperglycaemia, negative N_2 balance, lipolysis
   Supraphysiological doses are anti-inflammatory
3. Oestrogens, androgens (zona reticularis)
   Sex hormones

Adrenal medulla
Neural crest origin. Secretes catecholamines (from tyrosine):

1. Adrenalin
2. Noradrenalin
3. Dopamine
   Release stimulated by:
   Variety of stressful stimuli, e.g. pain, shock, endotoxin
   Actions: synergistic with other metabolically active
   hormones – prepare for 'flight or fight'
   Adrenergic receptors:
   Alpha:
   Vasoconstriction in most vascular beds except brain and heart
   Increased systolic, diastolic and mean blood pressure
   Beta:
   Vasodilatation and smooth muscle relaxation
   Mediate excitatory catecholamine effects on the heart-rate,
   output, and O_2 consumption
   $Beta_2$ receptors mediate metabolic actions

CUSHING'S SYNDROME

Causes
  1. Micropituitary adenomas – approx. 90%. Excess ACTH release,
     rarely CRF
  2. Adrenal adenoma or carcinoma – approx. 10%
  3. Ectopic ACTH production, 15%. Mostly from oat cell carcinoma
     of the lung, pancreatic islet cell carcinoma, thymic tumours.
     Patients with ectopic ACTH syndrome frequently do not appear
     Cushingoid, but have weakness, weight loss, and severe
     metabolic alkalosis
  4. Iatrogenic administration of corticosteroids is most common
     cause

Clinical manifestations
  1. Female : male 4 : 1
  2. Moon facies, buffalo hump, supraclavicular fat pad
  3. Purple striae
  4. Hypertension
  5. Hirsutism, acne
  6. Peripheral oedema
  7. Muscle wasting
  8. Osteoporosis
  9. Emotional lability, psychosis

Diagnostic tests
  1. 24-hour urinary free cortisol
  2. Dexamethasone suppression test
  3. Plasma ACTH level (elevated with pituitary causes)
  4. High dose dexamethasone suppression test

5. Metapyrone test
6. ACTH and CRF stimulation tests
7. Computed tomography of the adrenals, MRI brain

Treatment
1. Pituitary microdissection is treatment of choice for pituitary lesions
2. Radiation used infrequently
3. Neuropharmacological agents:
   Cyproheptadine blocks CRF
   Bromocriptine inhibits CRF secretion
4. Adrenalectomy: for adenoma/carcinoma if resectable
5. Mitotane. Chemotherapeutic agent for adrenal carcinoma

ADRENAL INSUFFICIENCY

Causes of acute insufficiency
1. Rapid withdrawal/failure or absorption of long-term steroid therapy. This is the most common cause
2. Haemorrhage into adrenals:
   Foetal distress
   Waterhouse–Friderichsen syndrome
   Anticoagulant therapy
   Post-delivery
   Post venography – adrenal vein thrombosis

Cause of chronic insufficiency
Autoimmune destruction of the adrenal glands

Clinical manifestations
1. Acute adrenal insufficiency:
   Fever; may be sudden and very high
   Nausea; very common
   Abdominal pain simulating bowel obstruction
   Lethargy
   Shock ensues if condition remains unrecognized
2. Chronic adrenal insufficiency
   Electrolyte abnormalities. Low serum Na^+, high K^+
   Weakness and weight loss
   Hyperpigmentation

CORTICOSTEROID THERAPY

Surgical complications
1. Masking of usual signs of peritonitis, e.g. fever, guarding
2. Retarded wound healing

3. Opportunistic postoperative infections, e.g. candida, especially with concomitant use of antibiotics
4. Potentiation of gastric ulcers
5. Pathological fractures
6. Reactivation of TB
7. Avascular necrosis (femoral head)
8. Cataracts

Perioperative management
1. Stress dose is hydrocortisone 100 mg 8-hourly
2. There is no reliable test of the hypothalamopituitary axis – therefore cover any patient who has been on steroids within 2 years of surgery. If in doubt cover the patient

CONN'S SYNDROME (PRIMARY HYPERALDOSTERONISM)

Clinical manifestations
1. Hypertension
2. Hypernatraemia, hypokalaemia, elevated bicarbonate
3. Weakness, tetany, polyuria, eclampsia of pregnancy, severe menorrhagia
4. Majority of cases are due to a unilateral adenoma

Diagnostic tests
1. CT/MRI of adrenal
2. Elevated serum aldosterone, and depressed renin, typical electrolyte changes

Treatment
1. Correction of hypokalaemia with potassium and spironolactone
2. Adrenalectomy

PHAEOCHROMOCYTOMA

Location
1. Adrenal medulla: 85–90%
   Bilateral in 10%
   Children 35–40%
   MEA 50%
   Malignant in 10%
2. Extra adrenal paraganglia
3. Organ of Zuckerkandl: this is a vestigial structure of chromaffin in the region of the aortic bifurcation
4. Bladder – can mostly be diagnosed by cystoscopy
5. Extra abdominal
   Brain

Neck

Thorax – almost always posteriorly

Clinical manifestations
1. Paroxysmal hypertension 50%
2. Headaches
3. Sweating and palpitations
4. Precipitated by anaesthesia, invasive tests, delivery etc.
5. Psychiatric changes

Diagnostic tests
1. Urinary or blood free catecholamines
2. MRI
3. MIBG scanning
4. Ultrasound of gallbladder to rule out associated gallstones

Associated conditions
1. MEA IIa
   Medullary thyroid carcinoma (MTC)
   Parathyroid hyperplasia
   Phaeochromocytoma frequently bilateral and multiple
2. MEA IIb
   MTC
   Parathyroid hyperplasia very rarely
   Mucosal neuromata, ganglioneuromatosis, characteristic
   phenotype
   Phaeochromocytoma
3. Von Recklinghausen's disease 1–2%
4. Von Hippel–Lindau disease
   Retinal angiomatosis
   Haemangioblastoma of cerebellum/spinal cord

Treatment
1. Alpha blockade (phenoxybenzamine) to counteract
   vasoconstriction and hypertension. Begins 2–3 weeks before
   operation
2. Volume replacement
3. Beta blockers for patients with tachycardias or arrhythmias, once
   alpha blockade is accomplished
4. Resection

THE INCIDENTALLY DISCOVERED ADRENAL MASS

1. Increasingly recognized as a result of increasing use of CT and
   MRI
2. Lesions less than 6 cm in size which are shown to be non-
   functional and do not increase in size over an 18–24 month
   period can be left alone

3. Lesions larger than 6 cm or lesions which are shown to have hormonal function are resected

30. Nervous system

CAUSES OF AN INTRACRANIAL MASS

1. Tumour
2. Haematoma
3. Abscess
4. Hydatid, TB, gumma – rare

FEATURES OF RAISED INTRACRANIAL PRESSURE

1. Headache – worse in morning and on coughing
2. Vomiting – often without nausea
3. Blurred vision
4. Mental deterioration and drowsiness
5. Increased head circumference – in newborn
6. Occurs early with posterior fossa and midline lesions, and late with frontal lesions
7. Papilloedema may not be present

MECHANISM OF INCREASED CSF PRESSURE

1. Mass effect within rigid cranium
2. Surrounding oedema
3. Block to circulation of CSF

BRAIN TUMOURS

Classification
1. Glioma – most common
    (i) Glioblastoma multiforme
    (ii) Astrocytoma
    (iii) Ependymoma
    (iv) Medulloblastoma
    (v) Oligodendroglioma
2. Meningioma
3. Neurilemmoma – acoustic neuroma

4. Pituitary tumours
5. Metastases
6. Rarer – craniopharyngioma, demoid, vascular tumours

Clinical features
1. Progressive focal neurological deficit
2. Late onset epilepsy
3. Dementia
4. Symptoms of raised intracranial pressure
5. History of primary carcinoma, e.g. bronchus/kidney
6. In children 70% of tumours are infratentorial
7. In adults 70% of tumours are supratentorial

COMMON SITES FOR MENINGIOMAS
1. Sphenoid ridge
2. Olfactory groove
3. Suprasellar region
4. Vault
5. Falx
6. Spinal canal

Pituitary tumour

Types
1. Chromophobe adenoma – most common – some secrete prolactin
2. Eosinophil adenoma – gigantism/acromegaly
3. Basophil adenoma – Cushing's syndrome

Complications
1. Bitemporal hemianopia
2. Hypopituitarism
3. Diabetes insipidus
4. Hormonal secretion

Acoustic neuroma
1. VIII nerve palsy – deafness, tinnitus, vertigo
2. VII nerve palsy – facial weakness, unilateral taste loss
3. V nerve palsy – facial numbness, loss of corneal reflex
4. IX, X, nerve palsy – dysphagia, hoarseness
5. Cerebellar syndrome
6. Raised intracranial pressure

CEREBRAL ABSCESS

Causes
1. Local spread from:

(i) Ear infection – esp. to temporal lobe and cerebellum
(ii) Sinus infection – esp. to frontal lobe
2. Blood spread, e.g. bronchiectasis, cyanotic congenital heart disease. May be multiple
3. Penetrating trauma

Clinical features
1. Needs to be differentiated from other space-occupying lesions, e.g. neoplasm, haematoma
2. May have an insidious or rapid onset
3. Systemic toxicity may be absent
4. Localizing signs may be absent or late in onset
5. May present years after the initiating infection

Management
1. Aspiration
2. Systemic and local antibiotics
3. Monitor abscess size with CT scan
4. Anticonvulsants
5. Late excision of scar sometimes stops seizures

SUBARACHNOID HAEMORRHAGE

Causes
1. Aneurysms 50%
2. Arteriovenous malformations 6%
3. Less common causes such as bleeding from tumours, eclampsia, anticoagulants, etc.
4. Idiopathic – remainder

Clinical features
1. Severe onset of headache, nausea, vomiting
2. Loss of consciousness may occur ± convulsions
3. 20% cases die within 24 hours of the first bleed
4. Ensuing sterile meningitis causes neck stiffness, photophobia
5. Stress may precipitate the bleed but 30% occur during sleep
6. Cerebral artery spasm may leed to further neurological damage in 35% patients
7. Recurrent bleeding
   (i) Rare in patients without aneurysms on angiography
   (ii) 20% of aneurysm cases within the first 2 weeks
   (iii) Carries a 50% mortality rate
   (iv) 5% rate in the first year following bleeding from an A-V malformation
8. Hydrocephalus

Management
1. Establish diagnosis by MRI/CT scan or presence of xanthochromia in the CSF
2. Early angiography to detect surgically correctable lesions
3. 2 weeks strict bed rest for those with no detectable lesion
4. Cases found to have an aneurysm require surgery. The timing of surgery is still subject of some debate. Early surgery reduces the risk of rebleeding and vasospasm, and has an increased morbidity because the brain is still oedematous, and the dissection more difficult. If surgery is postponed for 3 weeks the operation is easier but the risk of rebleeding and vasospasm in the interval is higher. If surgery is delayed, antifibrinolytic agents may be used to decrease rebleeding rate
5. Ventriculoperitoneal shunts may be required to treat hydrocephalus

INTRACRANIAL ANEURYSMS

Sites
Typically occur at vessel bifurcations
1. Junction of posterior communicating with internal carotid
2. Junction of anterior communicating with anterior cerebral
3. At first major branch of middle cerebral
4. Terminal bifurcation of the basilar artery
5. Multiple in 20%

Complications
1. Rupture more common with lesions > 5 mm
   (i) Subarachnoid haemorrhage
   (ii) Intracerebral haemorrhage
   (iii) Carotico-cavernous sinus fistula
2. Pressure. Prior to rupture, local pressure effect can cause:
   (i) Headache
   (ii) Cranial nerve palsy (III, IV, V, VI)

Clinical features
Commonly associated with:
1. Hypertension (Charcot's microaneurysms)
2. A-V malformations
3. Coagulopathy
4. Brain tumours

HEAD INJURY

Management
1. Ensure adequate airway

    (i) Oral airway
   (ii) Intubation – if patient cannot follow commands. Avoid neck flexion in case there is a cervical spine injury
2. Avoid hypotension
    (i) Scalp lacerations rarely bleed enough to cause hypotension
   (ii) Suspect intra-abdominal/thoracic bleeding/fracture-associated bleeding
3. Lower elevated intracranial pressure
    (i) Mechanical reduction
      a. Elevate head of bed
      b. Ventricular drain
      c. Evacuate haematoma
   (ii) Induce vasoconstriction
      a. Hyperventilation to reduce Pco^2
      b. i.v. bicarbonate
  (iii) Osmotic agents, e.g. mannitol
  (iv) Corticosteroids
   (v) Dehydration of brain with diuretics
4. Accurate initial neurological assessment of patient
    (i) Glasgow Coma Scale:
      a. Eye opening
      b. Best motor response
      c. Verbal response
   (ii) Duration of retrograde and antegrade amnesia
5. Head CT:
    (i) Change in level of consciousness
   (ii) Persistent lethargy
  (iii) Focal neurological signs
  (iv) Comatose patients
6. Cross-table lateral cervical spine X-rays with shoulders pulled down for clear view of C1–T1 alignment, in cases where spinal injury is suspected

Complications
1. Haemorrhage. (Any diminution in level of consciousness is assumed to be due to pressure from haematoma. However other causes, e.g., airway obstruction, intraperitoneal bleeding, must be excluded
   a. Epidural haematoma – most commonly from rupture of the middle meningeal artery and a fracture of the temporal bone
     (i) May present with lucid interval followed by deteriorating level of consciousness. This however is unusual
    (ii) May occur without a skull fracture especially in children
    (iii) Best seen on CT
    (iv) Rapid surgical decompression is required
   b. Subdural haematoma
     (i) Acute form generally associated with significant brain injury and may have arterial and venous bleeding

    (ii) Chronic form may be associated with cerebral atrophy, and trivial injury can initiate bleeding (venous)

    (iii) Signs of acutely expanding haematoma
      a. Diminution in level of consciousness
      b. Unilateral pupillary dilatation
      c. Systolic hypertension
      d. Bradycardia

2. Skull fracture
    (i) May be compound via skin/nose/ear. Patients with CSF leaks may require operative closure if leak persists for longer than 10 days
    (ii) Fragments may require elevation if depressed more than the thickness of the skull (1 cm), lie over a motor area, or if the fragment is sharp

3. Meningitis may follow compound injuries

4. Diabetes insipidus/inappropriate ADH release from pituitary damage

5. Hyperpyrexia – hypothalamic injury

6. Convulsions – esp. following long period of unconsciousness

7. Communicating hydrocephalus – weeks or months later

8. Psychological problems
    (i) Personality change
    (ii) Mood – depression
    (iii) Loss of memory, headaches, fatigue

9. Anosmia

10. Long-term severe cases require skin, bowel, catheter, nutritional care

SPINA BIFIDA

1. *Spina bifida occulta*
    (i) Usually asymptomatic
    (ii) Skin dimple, hair tuft, angioma may mark site in lumbar area
    (iii) Can be associated with a bony spur in spinal canal, causing enuresis, foot drop, backache. Excision of spur can be curative

2. *Dermal sinur tract*
    (i) May be hidden by hair
    (ii) May cause recurrent mixed flora meningitis
    (iii) Treated by excision

3. *Meningocoele*
    (i) Meninges protrude
    (ii) Should be excised and strong tissue brought over the lesion to prevent ulceration
    (iii) No neurological deficit

4. Myelomeningocoele and myelocoele
   (i) Mixed upper and lower motor neurone deficit
   (ii) Spincter disturbance
   (iii) Scoliosis, congenital dislocation of hips, talipes common
   (iv) Nearly all have hydrocephalus from Arnold Chiari
   malformation

Management
1. Conservative for those with poor prognosis
   (i) Flaccidity
   (ii) Severe hydrocephalus
   (iii) Multiple anomalies
2. Surgery
   (i) Closure of defect within first few hours of life to prevent
   infection
   (ii) Shunt for hydrocephalus if it develops
3. Orthopaedic and urological procedures later
4. Physiotherapy and special training

SPINAL CORD INJURIES

Clinical features
1. Patients may not have local pain or tenderness, leading to
   delayed diagnosis
2. X-rays may be poor quality
3. Attention may be diverted to other injuries
4. If in doubt immobilize

Complications
Injury is more common at junction of mobile and fixed portions of
vertebral column, e.g. lower cervical (50–60%), upper and lower
lumbar areas (20–30%)
1. Complete cord transection
   (i) Initial flaccid paralysis
   (ii) Initial arreflexia, later hyperreflexia
   (iii) Complete sensory loss below the lesion
   (iv) Sphincter denervation – urinary retention, faecal impaction
   (v) Hypotension – sympathectomy
   (vi) Priapism – useful diagnostic sign
2. Brown–Sequard syndrome (injury to lateral half of the cord)
   (i) Ipsilateral paralysis with loss of vibration and position
   (ii) Contralateral loss of pain and temperature sensation
3. Anterior spinal artery syndrome
   (i) Bilateral paralysis and loss of pain and temperature sensation
   (ii) Preservation of vibration and position sense
4. Cauda equina injury. Below L1
   Lower motor neurone lesion

Management
1. Immobilization
   (i) Four poster collar
   (ii) Crutchfield tongs
   (iii) Stryker frame
2. Decompression. Laminectomy in cases with spinal canal block indicated by progressive signs of compression and myelography/contrast CT. Surgery is rarely required or successful
3. In paraplegics care of:
   (i) Skin – pressure areas
   (ii) Bladder
   (iii) Bowels
   (iv) Fixation of unstable fractures
4. Rehabilitation

PROLAPSED INTERVERTEBRAL DISCS

Common sites
Usually occur posterolaterally
L4–L5   affects L5 root 80%
L5–S1   affects S1 root
C5–C6   affects C6 root 19%
C6–C7   affects C7 root

Clinical features
1. Pain
   a. Cervical disc – arm pain – interscapular pain
   b. Lumbar disc – back pain, sciatica, increased by straight leg raising
2. Weakness and atrophy of muscles
3. Diminished reflexes
4. Sensory loss
5. Local paravertebral muscle spasm and loss of lordosis
6. Central prolapse of disc may cause:
   (i) Sudden paralysis
   (ii) Sphincter disorder
   (iii) Bilateral sciatica

Localizing signs
1. L5
   (i) Weakness of ext. hall. longus
   (ii) Decreased sensation dorsum of foot
2. S1
   (i) Weakness of plantar flexion
   (ii) Ankle reflex loss
   (iii) Sensation decreased over lateral side of foot

3. C6
   (i) Weak biceps and wrist extensors
   (ii) Loss of biceps and brachioradialis reflex
   (iii) Sensory loss on thumb
4. C7
   (i) Weak triceps
   (ii) Triceps reflex decreased
   (iii) Sensory loss over middle finger

Indications for surgery
1. Central prolapse – emergency
2. Unremitting symptoms following conservative treatment, e.g. bed rest, traction
3. Severe neurological disturbance

Differential diagnosis of sciatica
1. Disc disease
2. Spinal tumour – primary or secondary
3. Intermittent claudication
4. Osteoarthrosis
5. Rectal and prostatic carcinoma. (Rectal examination must be done in all cases of sciatica)
6. Claudication of the cauda equina

EXTRADURAL SPINAL ABSCESS

Causes
1. Septicaemia
2. Osteomyelitis of the spine
3. Epidural anaesthetic

Clinical features
1. Pain
2. Tenderness
3. Fever
4. Paralysis

CAUSES OF SPINAL CORD COMPRESSION

1. Extradural
   (i) Metastases to spine
   (ii) Lymphoma, myeloma
   (iii) Disc, vertebral collapse, spondylosis
   (iv) TB, abscess
   (v) Haematoma

2. *Intradural extramedullary*
   (i) Meningioma
   (ii) Neurofibroma
   (iii) Archnoid cyst, etc. rare

3. *Intramedullary*
   (i) Glioma
   (ii) Syringo/haematomyelia

PERIPHERAL NERVE INJURIES

1. *Neuropraxia*
   (i) Axon and sheath intact
   (ii) Compression, e.g. tourniquet, crutch, plaster cast, or stretch, e.g. dislocations are common causes
   (iii) Good prognosis

2. *Axonotmesis*
   (i) Sheath intact
   (ii) Axonal disruption
   (iii) Axons regenerate 1 mm/day. Sensory function usually returns well. If site of injury is more than 40 cm from denervated muscle, then permanent muscle atrophy will occur by the time that reinnervation takes place

3. *Neurotmesis*
   (i) Sheath and axonal disruption
   (ii) Prognosis is better for pure motor or sensory nerves
   (iii) In mixed nerves cross innervation occurs
   (iv) Accurate opposition of severed ends is key factor

Management
   1. Maintain position of function
   2. Active or passive range of motion
   3. Surgery for neurotmesis with microscopic opposition
      a. Immediate for clean wounds
      b. Delayed for contaminated wounds
   4. Transposition/nerve interposition grafts sometimes required
   5. Tendon transfer for increased function
   6. Arthrodesis for unstable joints

Specific peripheral nerve injuries

1. *Erb's paralysis*
   C5, C6, injury after head is forced away from the shoulder, e.g. obstetric injury
      a. Motor deficit:

  (i) Loss of abduction and lateral rotation of the shoulder
  (ii) Loss of flexion and supination of the elbow
  (iii) Weakness of wrist extension
  b. Sensory deficit
  Upper outer shoulder

2. *Klumpke's paralysis*
   T1 injury, e.g. cervical rib, Pancoast tumour
   a. Motor deficit:
   Loss of intrinsic muscles of the hand except those supplied by
   the median nerve, i.e. abductor, opponens and fl. poll. brevis,
   and lateral two lumbricals
   b. Sensory deficit:
   Medial two fingers and medial forearm
   c. Horner's syndrome may be present

3. *Radial nerve*
   Crutch palsy, fracture of humerus
   a. Motor deficit:
   Wrist drop. Wrist extensor paralysis
   b. Sensory deficit:
   Very small area between the dorsum of thumb and index finger

4. *Median nerve*
   Elbow fractures, wrist lacerations, carpal tunnel syndrome
   a. Motor deficit:
      (i) Wrist level. Loss of thenar muscles except adductor poll;
          detected clinically by loss thumb abduction
      (ii) Elbow level. Loss of pronators of the forearm and digital
           flexors (except fl. c. ulnaris and fl. d. profundus to ring and
           little fingers) in addition to loss of thenar muscles as (i)
           above
   b. Sensory deficit:
      (i) Wrist level. Palmar aspects of thumb and lateral 2½ fingers
      (ii) Elbow level. Radial ⅔ of the palm as well as above.

5. *Ulnar nerve*
   Elbow or wrist injury
   a. Motor deficit:
      (i) Wrist level. Loss of all intrinsic hand muscles except those
          supplied by median nerve (see above)
      (ii) Elbow level. Loss of fl.c.uln., fl d. prof. to ring and little
           fingers, in addition to (i) above
   b. Sensory deficit:
      (i) Wrist level. Median 1½ fingers
      (ii) Elbow level. Medial palm as well as above

6. *Sciatic nerve*
   Posterior dislocation of the hip, penetrating wound
   a. Motor deficit:
      (i) Foot drop
      (ii) Loss of all movement below the knee
      (iii) Paralysis of the hamstrings
   b. Sensory deficit:
      Below the knee except for the area supplied by the long saphenous nerve

7. *Common peroneal nerve*
   Pressure from cast or stirrups in lithotomy position
   a. Motor deficit:
      (i) Foot drop
      (ii) Loss of eversion
   b. Sensory deficit:
      Anterior and lateral aspect of the foot

STROKE

Causes
1. Cardiac disorders
2. Atherosclerosis in cerebral vessels
3. Thromboembolism
   (i) Transient ischaemic attacks (TIA) – recovery in 1–7 hours. About ⅓ of patients will suffer complete stroke in 5 years if untreated
      a. Carotid disease
         (i) Amaurosis fugax
         (ii) Paralysis
         (iii) Dysphasia
         (iv) Hemisensory loss
      b. Vertebrobasilar disease
         (i) Homonymous field defect
         (ii) Diplopia
         (iii) Dysarthria
         (iv) Quadraparesis
         (v) Drop attacks
   (ii) Reversible ischaemic neurological deficits (RIND) recovery 1–7 days
   (iii) Infarction – fixed neurological deficit

Treatment
1. Medical management with aspirin or antiplatelet agents
2. Carotid endarterectomy
   (i) High grade stenoses
   (ii) Ulcerated plaques

(iii) Asymptomatic carotid disease – controversial

INTESTINAL ISCHAEMIA

Causes

Acute
1. Strangulated obstruction
2. Arterial embolus
3. Arterial thrombosis
4. Mesenteric venous thrombosis (hypercoagulable states)
5. Non-occlusive infarction. Follows a sustained decrease in cardiac output, e.g. hypovolaemia, myocardial infarction. Patients commonly on digoxin
6. Ischaemic colitis. Small vessel disease ranging in severity from gangrene to mild transient ischaemia with pain. Oral contraceptives implicated in some areas

Chronic
Intestinal angina
1. Post-prandial pain
2. Weight loss

Clinical features
1. Diagnosis often delayed
   (i) Mainly affects elderly patients
   (ii) Abdominal pain present to variable extent – may be absent
   (iii) Minimal findings on abdominal exam not unusual
2. Findings may include:
   (i) Bloody diarrhoea
   (ii) Signs of hypovolaemia (raised haematocrit)
   (iii) Ischaemic colon may be visible via sigmoidoscope

Treatment
1. Early diagnosis
2. Correction of generalized volume and perfusion problems
3. Surgery
   (i) Relief of strangulating mechanism
   (ii) Revascularization/embolectomy/bypass ± anticoagulation
   (iii) Resection of dead bowel
   (iv) Second-look operation after 24 hours in selected cases

INDEX